AF887678

Choose this not that

for

High Blood Pressure

by

Personal Remedies

Published by Simple Software Publishing.

Copyright © 2014 by Personal Remedies, LLC
5 Oregon Street
Georgetown, MA 01833 USA

Second Edition

ISBN-13: 978-0-9652457-1-5 ISBN-10: 0-9652457-1-3

Printed by CreateSpace.

All rights reserved, including the right of reproduction in whole or in part in any form whatsoever.

Choose this not that

for

High Blood Pressure

Inside this book, you will find a list of food items and easy to follow suggestions on how to improve your health through nutrition and the food choices you make every day.

Suggestions are provided for those with high blood pressure or those who are prone to develop this condition.

In addition, the book contains similar information for those who have one of the following common health conditions, risks or a diet preference along with high blood pressure:

- Alzheimer's disease
- Cancer risk
- Depression
- Diabetes (Type 2)
- Excess body weight or obesity
- Gout
- High cholesterol
- High triglycerides
- Stress
- Vitamin D deficiency
- Wish to follow DASH diet

Table of Contents

Important Notes

The purpose of this book is to provide helpful and informative material and to educate. It is in no way intended as substitute for medical advice. We recommend in all cases that you contact your personal doctor or health care provider before you embark upon any new diet or treatment of yourself.

This book is sold with the understanding that the publisher, the author and the distributor of this book are neither liable, nor have responsibility to any person or entity with respect to any loss, damage or injury which is incurred as a consequence, directly or indirectly, of the use or application of any of the contents of this book.

How to use this book

The guidelines presented on the following pages are for an adult male or female. They do not apply to children, pregnant women or breast feeding mothers.

Our suggestions are organized by food groups. Within each food group, **items are presented in a specific and deliberate order**. In the case of recommended items (those that could improve your health), the most helpful remedies or suggestions are presented first. In the case of items to avoid (those that could worsen your conditions), the most critical ones to avoid are listed first. The items that are suggested under Instead Choose, or items that are not included in the previous two lists, are likely to be neutral for your health (i.e., neither improve nor worsen your conditions) based on the information available to us at the time.

Unfortunately, health issues often come our way in groups of two or more. If we are obese or under stress, then chances are we are also at risk with a number of other health issues such as cancer, high blood pressure, or Vitamin D deficiency. If we have Vitamin D deficiency then chances are we either suffer from or have higher risk of getting Osteoporosis, Crohn's disease or kidney problems. Each health issue often results in other health complications, thus the need for looking at a combination of health concerns and risks when formulating our nutrition plans and lifestyle changes. It is for that reason, that we have included separate guidelines for those who might suffer from the most likely and common combinations of health issues related to the main health concern addressed by this book.

One of the factors that make *Choose this not that* series of publications different from all others available to you in the market is that we offer nutrition guidelines for likely COMBINATIONS of illnesses and risks that may be relevant to your situation. We also give you specific guidance by telling you exactly which fish, fruit, vegetable, nut ... is the best for you as well as listing the worst items. We give you an ordered list of food items within each food group, not just a food group.

We have listed alternative therapies and herbal medicines relevant (either helpful or harmful) to your condition. But it is beyond the scope of this book to provide specific guidelines on dosage or how to best benefit from these options. We encourage you to explore these alternatives with your natural health care provider.

Our approach in the *Choose this not that* series is to help people improve or combat their health issues through nutrition (i.e., consumption of food items that they can easily find in their local grocery store), exercise and lifestyle changes. We accomplish that through identification of those items that can improve your health, those that can worsen it, and those that play a neutral role. We trust that you can use this information to alter your diet and lifestyle choices to improve your health and wellbeing.

How we developed the content of this book

To provide specific and actionable information and guidance on food choices that you make every day and how they might impact your health, we had to quantify a relative level of goodness (or badness) for every individual food item in our database as they relate to each specific illness or health concern tracked in our system.

Most food and nutrition related research and publications in the U.S. are focused on vitamins, minerals, micro-nutrients, and substances such as cholesterol, fat and fiber. And to a lesser extent there are studies and data on herbal remedies, alternative and complementary medicine, and non-western treatments.

There is very little data or widely accepted studies that focus on individual foods (e.g., watermelon, white fish and walnuts) and how they relate to specific illnesses or health risks. Our goal has been to help address that void.

Here is a very brief description of our approach:

a) We maintain detailed nutrition information on every individual food item in our system. Most of such data is available from the U.S. Department of Agriculture. And for some data (e.g., Mercury, Gluten) we have found other reliable sources.

b) When there is data available on health benefits (or adverse impact) of a specific food item, or nutrient (e.g., vitamins, minerals) we capture and make use of such data.

c) If a given nutrient is good for a health condition (e.g., Vitamin A is good for night blindness), then all food items that are rich in that nutrient (Vitamin A) are given a positive/higher rating as they relate to that condition (night blindness). Similarly if a given nutrient has adverse impact on a health condition then all food items that contain that nutrient are given a negative/lower rating.

d) Some food items contain much more of a nutrient than others. Our technology takes that into account.

e) Some nutrients are found to be much more effective (e.g., Vitamin A) than some other nutrient (e.g., Zinc) as they relate to a given health condition (e.g., night blindness). Our technology distinguishes between the two.

f) Sometimes a study or a source behind the relationship between a nutrient and a health condition is much more reliable than another. Our approach is sensitive to that.

g) Certain nutrients facilitate absorption of another nutrient (e.g., Vitamin D facilitates absorption of Calcium). We make use of such information. For example, let's say Calcium is good for Tooth Development. Then all food items that are rich in Vitamin D are given a more positive consideration as they relate to Tooth Development.

h) Similarly some substances may reduce absorption of or increase the need for another (e.g., Caffeine may increase the need for Calcium). In the above example, all food items that contain Caffeine will receive a negative/lower rating as they relate to Tooth Development.

i) Our process and the steps mentioned above are automated by our unique (proprietary) and patented technology. At the conclusion of our process, there is a single score that represents the level of goodness or badness for every food item as it relates to each health condition maintained in our system. These scores are the basis for all the sorted lists of food items that you find in the Choose This Not That series of publications.

j) For multiple conditions, the sum of these scores is what drives the ranking of the food items and our guidelines.

In closing, it is important to note that in these publications we are not making scientific claims, nor do we suggest perfection of our approach. Our goal is to simply provide a significant improvement over status-quo. No human being or health care specialist can properly and fully take into account the enormity, complexity and contradictions inherent in the interrelationships of food, health, genetics, environment, exercise, lifestyle, etc. that affect our wellbeing. We have merely attempted to use the power of technology to provide you much better and more relevant information to maintain healthier living.

High Blood Pressure (HBP)

High blood pressure (HBP), also known as Hypertension, is a serious condition and can lead to other health issues such as heart attack, stroke and kidney failure.

Your blood pressure is an indication of how hard your heart has to work to pump blood through your arteries and how much resistance to blood flow exists in your arteries. It is highest when your heart beats, pumping the blood (systolic pressure). And it is the lowest between beats (diastolic pressure).

The blood pressure is often shown in form of a ratio, Systolic/Diastolic pressure, and measured in millimeters of mercury. Your blood pressure is considered normal if the Systolic number is less than 120 and Diastolic number is lower than 80. For example, if your blood pressure numbers are 115/79, you are fine. But if your top number is 140 or higher, or your bottom number is 90 or higher then you have HBP. If your numbers are in between normal and high, then you are likely to end up with HBP unless you take some action to prevent it.

There is no clear cause for HBP among adults. But there are some medical conditions (e.g., kidney problems, sleep apnea), certain medications (e.g., birth control pills) and use of some illegal drugs (e.g., cocaine) that can cause the blood pressure to rise.

You are more likely to develop HBP if you are: an over 55 man, an over 45 woman, black, overweight, physically inactive, under a lot of stress, smoke, drink too much alcohol, eat too much salt/sodium, do not eat enough potassium or Vitamin D, or have a family history of HBP.

Choose these for High Blood Pressure

Top 5 items to choose:

Garlic; Whole Grains; Soybeans; Seeds; Dried Fruits;

Food items and actions that could improve your health (within a food group, most helpful items are listed first):

Meat, Fish & Poultry

Pink salmon; Snail; Fish roe; Marlin; Swordfish; White fish; Trout; Carp; Snapper; Whelk; Sardines; Blue fin tuna; Mackerel; Ling; Sturgeon; Catfish; Seabass; Spot; Herring; Pollock; Monkfish; Tilefish; Halibut; Freshwater bass; Perch; Walleye; Bluefish; King mackerel; Pout; Smelt; Whiting; Striped bass; Yellowfin tuna; Pompano fish; Sheepshead; Yellowtail; Drum; Sucker; Wolffish; Cisco (smoked); Lingcod; Scup; Octopus; Caviar; Shad; Milkfish; Burbot; Cusk; Pumpkinseed sunfish; Shark; Eel; Mullet; Northern pike; Dolphinfish (Mahi-Mahi); Tilapia; Mussels; Rockfish; Surimi; Grouper; Cisco; Spiny lobster; Crayfish; Turbot; Calamari; Cuttlefish; Butterfish; Seatrout; Flatfish (flounder & sole); Beef brain; Dungeness crab; Beef liver; Oysters; Blue crab; Cod; Chicken breast (no skin); Haddock;

Eggs, Beans, Nuts and Seeds

Soybean seeds; Almonds; Hazelnuts or Filberts; Split peas; Seeds: breadnut tree, chia, cottonseed, flaxseed, safflower, sunflower; Soy milk; Soybeans (green); Breadfruit seeds; Pine nuts; Pistachio nuts; Brazil nuts; Beans: adzuki, navy; Watermelon seeds; Beans: moth beans, winged; Butternuts; various beans; Chickpeas; Lentils; Ginkgo nuts; Pili nuts; Pumpkin & squash seeds; Cashew nuts; Walnuts; Peanuts; Chestnuts; Black-eyed peas; Green peas; Alfalfa sprouts; Lupin; Sugar or snap peas; Hickory nuts; Beechnuts; Sesame seeds; Acorns; Pecans; Cornnuts; Macadamia nuts

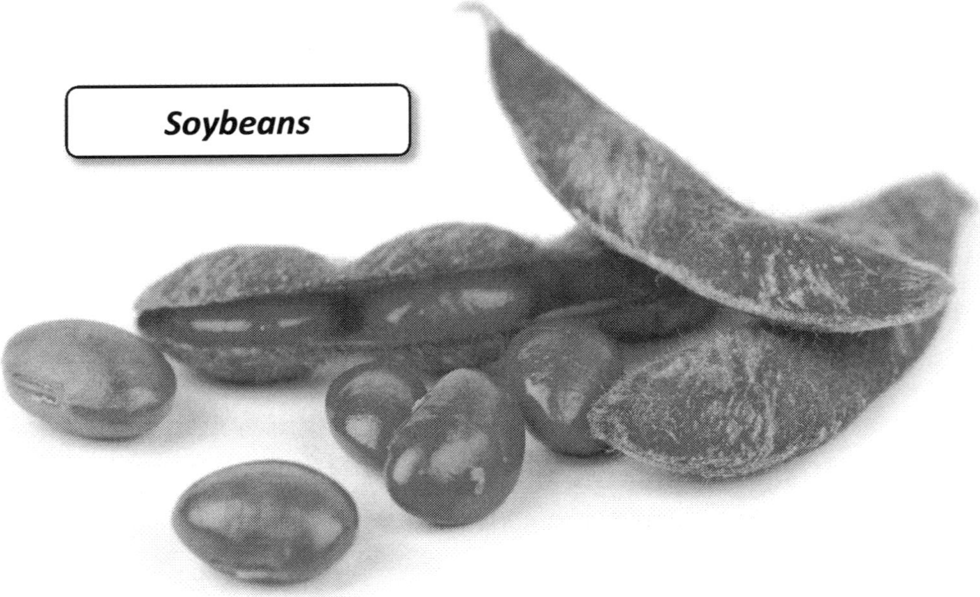

Fruits & Juices

Dried Fruits, especially: banana, litchi, prunes, raisins, figs, peaches, apricots, currants; Tamarind; Goji berries; Dates; Passion fruit; Prune juice; Grape juice; Banana; Abiyuch; Elderberries; Guava; Pineapple juice; Plantains; Cranberry juice; Breadfruit; Currants (raw); Durian; Kiwi fruit; Avocado; Pears; Apricots; Blackberries; Boysenberries; Cantaloupe; Jujube (fruit); Kumquats; Loganberry; Longans; Natal Plum (Carissa); Persimmons; Raspberries; Rowal; Apple juice; Grapefruit juice; Orange juice; Figs; various berries; Lemon; Lime; Pomegranate; Apples; Grapes; Peaches; Acerola; Cherries; Grapefruit; Honeydew melon; Litchi; Mango; Nectarine; Oranges; Papaya; Pineapple; Pitanga; Plum; Pomegranate juice; Pumelo (Shaddock); Quince; Strawberries; Tangerines; Watermelon;

Vegetables

Garlic; Amaranth leaves; Epazote; Fungi cloud ears; Grape leaves; Shitake mushrooms; Peppers: ancho, pasilla; Pigeon peas; Sun-dried tomatoes; Wasabi root; Arrowhead; Taro leaves; Balsam pear leafy tips; Corn bran; Sweet potatoes leaves; Tahitian taro; Vine spinach (Basella); Artichoke; Chrysanthemum (Garland); Chrysanthemum Leaves; Dandelion Greens; Mustard spinach; Garden cress; Kale; Potatoes w/skin; Arugula; Kelp; Nopal; Taro; Chinese broccoli; Chicory greens; Collards; Mustard greens; Okra; Turnip greens; Yam; Quinoa seed; Bok choy; Borage; Cowpeas leafy tips; Purslane; Watercress; Winged beans leaves; Lotus root; Onions (2-5 oz. of fresh onion daily, or 1 tsp. onion juice 3-4 times a day); Parsnips; Cauliflower; Beet greens; Balsam pear; Broccoli; Brussels sprouts; Carrots; Endive; Fiddlehead ferns; Green onions (scallions); Kohlrabi; Shallots; Arrowroot; Jerusalem artichoke; Portabella mushrooms; Beets; Celtuce; Hot chili peppers; Rutabaga; Spinach; Squash: winter, yellow; Zucchini; Lambsquarters; various cabbage; Eggplant; Green beans; various peppers; Corn; Potato; Asparagus; Bell peppers; Cucumbers with peel; Leeks; various lettuce; other vegetables;

Breads, Grains, Cereals, Pasta

Wheat bran; Wheat germ; Whole-wheat; Amaranth; Whole-wheat bread; Buckwheat; Wheat germ cereal; Durum wheat; Oats; Rye; Whole-wheat English muffins; Whole-wheat cereal; Triticale; Rice bran; Whole-wheat spaghetti; Sorghum; Wheat germ bread; Bran flakes cereal; Wheat bran muffins; Oatmeal (cereal); Spelt (cooked); Oat bran muffins; Millet; Brown rice; Shredded wheat cereal; Whole-wheat dinner rolls; Barley; Bulgur; Wild rice; Granola cereal; Rice cakes (Brown rice based); Tortillas (corn); Whole-wheat crackers; Oat bran bread; Oat bran; Semolina; Pumpernickel bread;

Dairy Products, Fats & Oils

Whey (dried); Wheat germ oil; Cheese: Gjetost, cottage, Swiss; Cod liver fish oil; Flaxseed oil; various fish oil; Gruyere cheese; Chocolate milk; Fat-free or Low Fat products;

Desserts, Snacks, Beverages

Sesame crunch candies; Molasses; Air popped popcorn; Dark chocolate; Red wine; White wine; Peanut butter; Water; Hot chocolate; Tonic water;

Herbs & Spices, Fast Foods, Prepared Foods

Whole-grain cornmeal; Cottonseed meal; Thyme (fresh); Tofu; Peppermint; Natto; Rosemary (fresh); Cheese fondue; Tempeh; Parsley; Dill weed; Spearmint (fresh); Sorghum syrup; Basil (fresh); Cocoa; Tarragon (dried); Succotash; French fries; Coriander/Cilantro; Fennel seeds; Oregano; Sage; Tomato paste; Chervil; Poppy seed; Pepper (black or white);Cinnamon; Cayenne (red) pepper;

Alternative Therapies & Miscellaneous

Follow DASH diet; Exercise; Fresh (uncooked) fruits/veg's or use no salt added cans; Meditation; Ornish Plan & Diet; Pray, practice your religion; Sleep 6-8 hours regularly; Tai Chi; Yoga (avoid certain postures); Salt-free or low-salt foods; Organically grown foods; 1-2 alcoholic drinks/day; Biofeedback; Exposure to sun; Hypnotherapy; Laugh, laughter; Sound Therapy; Vegetarian diet;

Key Nutrients & Herbal Medicines

Hawthorn (in berries form or tea from dried leaves and flowers. Do not take with other heart medications); Calcium; Celery seed; Siberian Ginseng; Magnesium; Potassium; Yucca; Barberry; Fiber; Kudzu; Lemon grass; Motherwort; Omega-3 fatty acids; Vitamin D;

Do not choose these for High Blood Pressure

Top 5 items to avoid:

2+ alcoholic drinks/day; Luncheon Meats; Sweets; Margarine & Hydrogenated vegetable oil; Table salt; & Excess Body Weight

Avoid or consume much less of the following (within a food group, most harmful items are listed first):

Meat, Fish & Poultry

Luncheon (processed) meats; Chorizo; Frankfurters; Pepperoni; Pork liver cheese; Pork skins; Salami; Sausage; Bacon; Cured meats; Pastrami; Beef jerky sticks; Bologna; Chicken skin; Turkey skins; Meatless sausage; Corned beef; Pork cured/ham; Pork headcheese; Salmon (smoked, Lox); Beef chuck/brisket; Beef tongue; Lamb tongue; Squab (pigeon); Beef ribs; Pork ribs; Lamb ribs; Beef shank; Chicken dark meat; Chicken wings; Pork spare ribs; Lamb loin; Lamb, ground; Pork back ribs; Goose; Bison/buffalo meat;

Instead choose: Canned tuna; Orange roughy; Scallops; Sablefish; Anchovy; Pork loin/sirloin; Venison; Turkey breast; Rabbit meat; White fish (smoked); Veal shank; Veal liver; Turkey dark meat; Boar meat; Beef filet mignon; Beef round steak; Veal; Duck (no skin); Quail breast;

Eggs, Beans, Nuts and Seeds

Coconut Milk;

Instead choose: Coconut meat (dried); Coconut; Egg white; Egg; Egg yolk;

Breads, Grains, Cereals, Pasta

Saltines crackers; Croissant; Danish pastry; Sweet cinnamon rolls; Wheat crackers; Rice crisps cereal; Kaiser dinner rolls; Milk crackers; Donuts; French rolls; White bread; Sweet rolls; Biscuits; Chinese chow Mein noodles; Hamburger & hot dog rolls; Bread sticks; Bagels; Blueberry muffins; Melba toasts crackers; Corn flakes cereal; Waffles;

Instead choose: Pumpernickel bread; Spinach spaghetti; White rice; Oat bran rolls; Wheat; Corn muffins; Cornbread; Egg noodles; Corn cakes; Spaghetti; Pasta; Rice noodles; Japanese noodles; Italian bread; Banana bread; Cream of wheat cereal; English muffins;

Dairy Products, Fats & Oils

Margarine (salted); Margarine-like spreads; Hydrogenated vegetable oil; Margarine (unsalted); Butter (salted); Animal fat; Oil: Babassu, Cocoa Butter, cottonseed, Cupu Assu, palm, peanut, poppy see, rice bran, sesame, Shea nut, tea seed, Ucuhuba Butter; Brie cheese; Lard; various nuts/seeds/veg oils; Vegetable shortening; Poultry fat; Cheese: Roquefort, goat, pimento, feta, camembert; Butter (unsalted); various cheese; Whipped cream; Cream; Sour cream; Non-dairy creamers;

Instead choose: Milk; Yogurt; Cheddar cheese; Ricotta cheese; Colby cheese;

Desserts, Snacks, Beverages

Pound cake; Sweet chocolate; various cookies; Puff pastry; Pie crust; Chocolate cake; Éclairs; Cheesecake; various cakes; Cream puffs; Pretzels; Dessert toppings; Coffeecake; Vanilla cream pie; Coffee liqueur; Chocolate mousse; Pecan pie; various pies; Coffee; Fruit leather/rolls; After-dinner mints; Ice cream; Peanut brittle candy; Pudding; Frostings; Ice cream cones; Potato sticks; Fruit punch; Lemonade; Soft (carbonated) drinks; Honey; Pancakes; Chewing gum; Jams & Preserves; Sherbet; Tea; various candies;

Instead choose: Potato chips/fried snacks; Sports drinks; Beer; Milk shakes; Halvah candies; Malted drinks (nonalcoholic); Eggnog; Tortilla chips; Applesauce; Crème de menthe; Ginger ale; Piña colada; Herbal tea; Jellies

Herbs & Spices, Fast Foods, Prepared Foods

Salad dressings: blue/Roquefort, French; Table salt; Oyster sauce; Italian salad dressing; Foie gras or liver pate; Sauces: Hoisin, Sofrito, barbecue; Hot dog; Capers; Mayonnaise; Cheese sauce; Breaded shrimp; Table sugar (white or powder); Soy sauce; Chicken Nuggets; Chocolate syrup; Nachos; Ketchup; Pizza; Tabasco sauce; Onion rings; Fish sauce; Hash brown potatoes; Syrup (table blends); Pickle relish; Mustard; Pickle (cucumber); Gravies (canned); Cheeseburger; Maple syrup; Macaroni; Tapioca; Potato salad; Sauerkraut; Croutons; Beef broth; Chicken broth; Chicken noodle soup; Veg/beef soup; Potato pancakes;

Instead choose: Mustard seed; Falafel; Miso; Saffron; Mints; Corn salad; Fish stock; Mace; Cardamom; Cloves; Chives; Couscous; Ginger; Marjoram; Brown sugar; Vinegar; Clam chowder; Nutmeg; Minestrone soup; Chicken stock; Beef stock;

Alternative Therapies & Miscellaneous

2+ alcoholic drinks/day; Excess body weight; Hyperthermia (avoid if extremely high blood pressure); Smoking, tobacco; Stress; Salted foods, nuts, etc.; Corn sweetener; Sugared fruit juice or from concentrate; Canned foods; Processed or Refined foods;

Key Nutrients & Herbal Medicines

Caffeine; Licorice; Sodium/salt (limit to 1,500 mg per day); Saturated fat; Total fat; Asian Ginseng; Refined sugar;

Food Look-up Table for HBP

Food Item or Other	Suitability for HBP	Remarks (if any)
1-2 alcoholic drinks/day	Helpful	
2+ alcoholic drinks/day	Avoid	
80+ proof distilled alc. bev.	Neutral/OK	
Abalone	Neutral/OK	
Abiyuch	More helpful	
Acerola	More helpful	
Acorns	More helpful	
After-dinner mints	Consume much less	
Alfalfa sprouts	More helpful	
Almonds	Most helpful	
Amaranth	Most helpful	
Amaranth leaves	Most helpful	
Anchovy	Helpful	
Apple juice	More helpful	
Apples	More helpful	
Apples, dried	More helpful	
Applesauce	Neutral/OK	
Apricots	More helpful	
Apricots, dried	Most helpful	
Arrowhead	Most helpful	
Arrowroot	More helpful	
Artichoke	Most helpful	
Artichoke, Jerusalem	More helpful	
Arugula	Most helpful	
Asparagus	More helpful	
Aspirin	Consume less	
Avocado	More helpful	
Bacon	Avoid	
Bagels	Consume less	
Balsam pear	More helpful	
Balsam pear leafy tips	Most helpful	
Banana	More helpful	
Banana, dried	Most helpful	
Barberry	Helpful	
Barley	More helpful	
Basil (fresh)	Helpful	
Bass, freshwater	More helpful	
Bass, Seabass	More helpful	
Bass, striped	More helpful	
Beans, adzuki	Most helpful	
Beans, baked	Most helpful	
Beans, black	Most helpful	
Beans, black-eyed peas	More helpful	
Beans, fava	Most helpful	
Beans, hyacinth	Most helpful	
Beans, kidney	Most helpful	
Beans, lima	More helpful	
Beans, moth beans	Most helpful	

Food Item or Other	Suitability for HBP	Remarks (if any)
Beans, Mung	Most helpful	
Beans, navy	Most helpful	
Beans, pinto	Most helpful	
Beans, winged	Most helpful	
Beans, Yardlong	Most helpful	
Beans, yel & white	Most helpful	
Bear meat	Neutral/OK	
Beaver meat	Neutral/OK	
Beechnuts	More helpful	
Beef brain	Helpful	
Beef chuck/brisket	Consume much less	
Beef filet mignon	Helpful	
Beef heart	Neutral/OK	
Beef jerky sticks	Avoid	
Beef kidneys	Neutral/OK	
Beef liver	Helpful	
Beef rib eye	Neutral/OK	
Beef ribs	Consume less	
Beef round steak	Neutral/OK	
Beef shank	Consume less	
Beef spleen	Helpful	
Beef tenderloin/Tbone/portrhse	Consume less	
Beef tongue	Consume less	
Beef top sirloin	Consume less	
Beef, cured breakfast strips	Avoid	
Beef, cured dried	Consume much less	
Beef, ground	Neutral/OK	
Beer	Helpful	
Beerwurst beer salami	Avoid	
Beet greens	More helpful	
Beets	More helpful	
Bell peppers, green	More helpful	
Bell peppers, red	More helpful	
Biofeedback	Helpful	
Birth control pills	Consume less	
Biscuits	Consume less	
Bison/buffalo meat	Consume less	
Blackberries	More helpful	
Blueberries and Bilberries	More helpful	
Bluefish	More helpful	
Boar meat	Helpful	
Bok choy	More helpful	
Bologna, various	Consume much less	
Borage	More helpful	
Boron	Helpful	
Boysenberries	More helpful	
Brazil nuts	Most helpful	
Bread sticks	Consume less	
Bread, banana	Neutral/OK	
Bread, cornbread	Neutral/OK	
Bread, Italian	Neutral/OK	

Food Item or Other	Suitability for HBP	Remarks (if any)
Bread, oat bran	Helpful	
Bread, oat bran, rolls	Helpful	
Bread, pumpernickel	Helpful	
Bread, wheat germ	Most helpful	
Bread, white	Consume less	
Bread, whole-wheat	Most helpful	
Breadfruit	More helpful	
Breadfruit seeds	Most helpful	
Broccoli	More helpful	
Broccoli, Chinese	Most helpful	
Brussels sprouts	More helpful	
Buckwheat	Most helpful	
Bulgur	More helpful	
Burbot	More helpful	
Butter (salted)	Avoid	
Butter (unsalted)	Consume much less	
Butterfish	Helpful	
Butternuts	Most helpful	
Cabbage, green	More helpful	
Cabbage, red	More helpful	
Cabbage, savoy	More helpful	
Caffeine	Consume much less	
Cake, angel food	Consume much less	
Cake, Boston cream pie	Avoid	
Cake, chocolate	Avoid	
Cake, gingerbread	Consume much less	
Cake, pound	Avoid	
Cake, shortcake	Consume much less	
Cake, sponge	Avoid	
Cake, yellow	Avoid	
Calamari	Helpful	
Calcium	More helpful	
Candies, caramels	Consume less	
Candies, carob	Consume less	
Candies, halvah	Neutral/OK	
Candies, hard	Consume less	
Candies, marshmallows	Consume less	
Candies, peanut bar	Consume less	
Candies, peanut brittle	Consume much less	
Candies, sesame crunch	Most helpful	
Candies, sweet chocolate	Avoid	
Canned foods	Consume less	
Cantaloupe	More helpful	
Capers	Consume much less	
Cardamom	Neutral/OK	
Caribou meat	Helpful	
Carp	Most helpful	
Carrots	More helpful	
Cashew nuts	Most helpful	
Catfish	More helpful	
Cauliflower	More helpful	

Food Item or Other	Suitability for HBP	Remarks (if any)
Caviar	More helpful	
Cayenne (red) pepper	Helpful	
Celery	Helpful	
Celery seed	More helpful	
Celtuce	More helpful	
Cereal, bran flakes	Most helpful	
Cereal, corn flakes	Consume less	
Cereal, cream of wheat	Consume less	
Cereal, granola	More helpful	
Cereal, rice crisps	Consume much less	
Cereal, shredded wheat	More helpful	
Cereal, wheat germ	Most helpful	
Cereal, whole-wheat	Most helpful	
Cheese fondue	More helpful	
Cheese spread	Consume much less	
Cheese, American	Consume much less	
Cheese, blue	Consume much less	
Cheese, Brie	Consume much less	
Cheese, camembert	Consume much less	
Cheese, cheddar	Neutral/OK	
Cheese, Colby	Consume less	
Cheese, cottage	Helpful	
Cheese, cream	Consume much less	
Cheese, edam	Consume less	
Cheese, feta	Consume much less	
Cheese, Fontina	Consume less	
Cheese, Gjetost	Helpful	
Cheese, goat	Consume much less	
Cheese, gouda	Consume less	
Cheese, gruyere	Helpful	
Cheese, limburger	Consume much less	
Cheese, mozzarella	Consume less	
Cheese, parmesan	Consume much less	
Cheese, pimento	Consume much less	
Cheese, port de salut	Consume less	
Cheese, ricotta	Neutral/OK	
Cheese, Romano	Consume less	
Cheese, Roquefort	Consume much less	
Cheese, Swiss	Helpful	
Cheeseburger	Consume less	
Cheesecake	Avoid	
Cherries	More helpful	
Chervil	Helpful	
Chestnuts	More helpful	
Chewing gum	Consume less	
Chicken breast (no skin)	Helpful	
Chicken dark meat	Consume less	
Chicken giblets	Neutral/OK	
Chicken heart	Consume less	
Chicken liver	Helpful	
Chicken Nuggets	Consume much less	

Food Item or Other	Suitability for HBP	Remarks (if any)
Chicken skin	Consume much less	
Chicken wings	Consume less	
Chickpeas	Most helpful	
Chicory greens	Most helpful	
Chives	Neutral/OK	
Chocolate mousse	Consume much less	
Chocolate, dark	Helpful	
Chorizo	Avoid	
Chrysanthemum (Garland)	Most helpful	
Chrysanthemum Leaves	Most helpful	
Cinnamon	Helpful	
Cisco	Helpful	
Cisco (smoked)	More helpful	
Clams	Consume less	
Cloves	Neutral/OK	
Cocoa	Helpful	
Coconut	Neutral/OK	
Coconut meat (dried)	Helpful	
Coconut milk	Consume less	
Cod	Helpful	
Coffee	Consume much less	
Coffee liqueur	Consume much less	
Coffeecake	Consume much less	
Collards	Most helpful	
Consult your doctor	Most helpful	
Cookies, animal crackers	Avoid	
Cookies, brownies	Avoid	
Cookies, butter	Avoid	
Cookies, chocolate chip	Avoid	
Cookies, gingersnaps	Consume much less	
Cookies, lady fingers	Consume much less	
Cookies, molasses	Consume much less	
Cookies, oatmeal	Consume much less	
Cookies, peanut butter	Avoid	
Cookies, shortbread	Avoid	
Cookies, sugar	Avoid	
Cookies, vanilla wafers	Avoid	
Coriander/Cilantro	Helpful	
Corn	More helpful	
Corn bran	Most helpful	
Corn cakes	Neutral/OK	
Corn salad	Helpful	
Corn sweetener	Consume less	
Corned beef	Consume much less	
Cornmeal, whole-grain	Most helpful	
Cornnuts	Helpful	
Cottonseed meal	Most helpful	
Couscous	Neutral/OK	
Cowberries	More helpful	
Cowpeas leafy tips	More helpful	
Crab, Alaskan King	Neutral/OK	

Food Item or Other	Suitability for HBP	Remarks (if any)
Crab, blue	Helpful	
Crab, Dungeness	Helpful	
Crackers, matzo	Consume less	
Crackers, melba toasts	Consume less	
Crackers, milk	Consume much less	
Crackers, saltines	Avoid	
Crackers, wheat	Consume much less	
Crackers, whole-wheat	Helpful	
Cranberries	Helpful	
Cranberry juice	More helpful	
Crayfish	Helpful	
Cream	Consume less	
Cream puffs	Avoid	
Cream, whipped	Consume much less	
Crème de menthe	Neutral/OK	
Croaker	Neutral/OK	
Croissant	Avoid	
Croutons	Consume less	
Cucumbers with peel	More helpful	
Cured meats	Avoid	
Currants (dried)	Most helpful	
Currants (raw)	More helpful	
Cusk	More helpful	
Cuttlefish	Helpful	
Dandelion Greens	Most helpful	
Danish pastry	Consume much less	
Dates	Most helpful	
Dessert toppings	Avoid	
Dill weed	More helpful	
Dolphinfish (Mahi-Mahi)	More helpful	
Donuts	Consume much less	
Drum	More helpful	
Duck (no skin)	Neutral/OK	
Durian	More helpful	
Durum wheat	Most helpful	
Éclairs	Avoid	
Eel	More helpful	
Egg (raw)	Neutral/OK	
Egg rolls (veg)	Consume less	
Egg substitute	Consume less	
Egg white	Neutral/OK	
Egg yolk	Neutral/OK	
Egg, boiled & poached	Neutral/OK	
Egg, duck & goose	Consume less	
Eggnog	Neutral/OK	
Eggplant	More helpful	
Elderberries	More helpful	
Endive	More helpful	
English muffins	Consume less	
English muffins, whole-wheat	Most helpful	
Epazote	Most helpful	

Food Item or Other	Suitability for HBP	Remarks (if any)
Excess body weight	Avoid	
Exercise	More helpful	
Exercise - cardiovascular	More helpful	
Exercise - weight training	More helpful	
Exposure to sun	Helpful	
Falafel	Helpful	
Fat, beef/lamb/pork	Consume much less	
Fat, chicken	Consume much less	
Fat, goose/duck	Consume much less	
Fat, saturated	Consume less	
Fat, total	Consume less	
Fat, turkey	Consume much less	
Fat-free or low fat products	More helpful	such as dairy products
Fennel	Helpful	
Fennel seeds	Helpful	
Fenugreek seeds	Helpful	
Fiber	Helpful	
Fiddlehead ferns	More helpful	
Figs	More helpful	
Figs, dried	Most helpful	
Fish oil, cod liver	Helpful	
Fish oil, herring	Helpful	
Fish oil, menhaden	Helpful	
Fish oil, salmon	Helpful	
Fish oil, sardine	Helpful	
Fish roe	Most helpful	
Flatfish (flounder & sole)	Helpful	
Fluoride	Helpful	
Foie gras or liver pate	Avoid	
Follow DASH diet	Most helpful	see separate chapter
Food prep -- fried or battered	Consume less	
Frankfurter, beef and pork	Avoid	
Frankfurter, chicken & turkey	Avoid	
French fries	Helpful	
French toast	Consume less	
Fresh (uncooked) fruits/veg's	More helpful	or use no salt added canned
Frostings	Consume less	
Frozen yogurt	Consume less	
Fruit juice, sugared/concentrate	Consume less	
Fruit leather/rolls	Consume much less	
Fruit punch	Consume less	
Fungi cloud ears	Most helpful	
Garden cress	Most helpful	
Garlic	Most helpful	
Ginger	Neutral/OK	
Ginger ale	Neutral/OK	
Ginkgo nuts	Most helpful	
Ginseng, Asian	Consume less	
Ginseng, Siberian	More helpful	
Goji berry	Most helpful	
Goose	Consume less	

Food Item or Other	Suitability for HBP	Remarks (if any)
Gooseberries	More helpful	
Granola bars	Consume less	
Grape juice	More helpful	
Grape leaves	Most helpful	
Grapefruit	More helpful	
Grapefruit juice	More helpful	
Grapes	More helpful	
Gravies (canned)	Consume less	
Green beans	More helpful	
Green onions (scallions)	More helpful	
Grouper	Helpful	
Guarana	Consume less	
Guava	More helpful	
Guinea hen	Neutral/OK	
Haddock	Helpful	
Halibut	More helpful	
Hamburger	Consume less	
Hash brown potatoes	Consume much less	
Hawthorn; Most helpful; in berries form or tea from dried leaves/flowers. Don't take with other heart medications.		
Hazelnuts or Filberts	Most helpful	
Hearts of palm	More helpful	
Herring	More helpful	
Hickory nuts	More helpful	
Honey	Consume less	
Honeydew melon	More helpful	
Horseradish	Consume less	
Hot chocolate	Consume less	
Hot dog	Avoid	
Hummus	Consume less	
Hush puppies	Consume less	
Hyperthermia	Consume much less	avoid if extremely high blood pressure
Hypnotherapy	Helpful	
Ice cream cones	Consume less	
Ice cream, chocolate	Avoid	
Ice cream, vanilla	Consume much less	
Jams & Preserves	Consume less	
Jellies	Consume less	
Jujube (fruit)	More helpful	
Kale	Most helpful	
Kelp	Most helpful	
Ketchup	Consume much less	
Kiwi fruit	More helpful	
Kohlrabi	More helpful	
Kola (cola)	Consume less	
Kudzu	Helpful	
Kumquats	More helpful	
Lamb brain	Helpful	
Lamb heart	Consume less	
Lamb kidneys	Neutral/OK	
Lamb leg	Neutral/OK	
Lamb liver	Neutral/OK	

Food Item or Other	Suitability for HBP	Remarks (if any)
Lamb loin	Consume less	
Lamb ribs	Consume less	
Lamb shoulder	Consume less	
Lamb spleen	Neutral/OK	
Lamb tongue	Consume less	
Lamb, ground	Consume less	
Lambsquarters	More helpful	
Lard	Consume much less	
Laugh, laughter	Helpful	
Leeks	More helpful	
Lemon	More helpful	
Lemon grass	Helpful	
Lemonade	Consume less	
Lentils	Most helpful	
Lettuce, cos or Romaine	More helpful	
Lettuce, head	More helpful	
Lettuce, loose leaf	More helpful	
Licorice	Consume much less	
Lime	More helpful	
Ling	More helpful	
Lingcod	More helpful	
Litchi	More helpful	
Litchi, dried	Most helpful	
Lobster	Neutral/OK	
Lobster, spiny	Helpful	
Loganberry	More helpful	
Longans	More helpful	
Longans, dried	Most helpful	
Lotus root	More helpful	
Luncheon meat, beef & pork	Avoid	
Luncheon meat, cured beef	Avoid	
Lupin	More helpful	
Macadamia nuts	Helpful	
Macaroni	Consume less	
Mace	Neutral/OK	
Mackerel	Most helpful	
Mackerel, king	More helpful	
Magnesium	More helpful	
Malted drinks (nonalcoholic)	Neutral/OK	
Mango	More helpful	
Margarine (salted)	Avoid	
Margarine (unsalted)	Avoid	
Margarine-like spreads	Avoid	
Marjoram	Neutral/OK	
Marlin	Most helpful	
Mate	Consume less	
Mayonnaise	Consume much less	
Meditation	More helpful	
Milk shakes	Helpful	
Milk, 2% fat	Helpful	
Milk, chocolate	Consume much less	

Food Item or Other	Suitability for HBP	Remarks (if any)
Milk, low fat (1%)	Helpful	
Milk, Skim milk	Helpful	
Milk, Whole milk	Helpful	
Milkfish	More helpful	
Millet	More helpful	
Mints	Helpful	
Miso	Helpful	
Molasses	Most helpful	
Molasses, blackstrap	Most helpful	
Monkfish	More helpful	
Motherwort	Helpful	
Muffins, blueberry	Consume less	
Muffins, corn	Helpful	
Muffins, oat bran	More helpful	
Muffins, wheat bran	Most helpful	
Mulberries	More helpful	
Mullet	More helpful	
Mushrooms, Jew's ear	More helpful	
Mushrooms, portabella	More helpful	
Mushrooms, shitake	Most helpful	
Mussels	Helpful	
Mustard	Consume less	
Mustard greens	Most helpful	
Mustard seed	Helpful	
Mustard spinach	Most helpful	
Nachos	Consume much less	
Natal Plum (Carissa)	More helpful	
Natto	Most helpful	
Nectarine	More helpful	
Non-dairy creamers	Consume less	
Noodles, Chinese chow Mein	Consume less	
Noodles, egg	Neutral/OK	
Noodles, Japanese	Neutral/OK	
Noodles, rice	Neutral/OK	
Nopal	Most helpful	
Nutmeg	Neutral/OK	
Oat bran	Helpful	
Oatmeal (cereal)	Most helpful	
Oats	Most helpful	
Octopus	More helpful	
Oil, almonds	Consume much less	
Oil, apricot kernel	Consume much less	
Oil, avocado	Consume much less	
Oil, Babassu	Consume much less	
Oil, canola	Consume less	
Oil, Cocoa Butter	Consume much less	
Oil, coconut	Consume much less	
Oil, corn	Consume much less	
Oil, cottonseed	Consume much less	
Oil, Cupu Assu	Consume much less	
Oil, flaxseed	Helpful	

Food Item or Other	Suitability for HBP	Remarks (if any)
Oil, grape seeds	Consume much less	
Oil, hazelnut	Consume much less	
Oil, hydrogenated vegetable	Avoid	
Oil, mustard	Consume much less	
Oil, oat	Consume much less	
Oil, olive	Consume much less	
Oil, palm	Consume much less	
Oil, peanut	Consume much less	
Oil, poppy seed	Consume much less	
Oil, rice bran	Consume much less	
Oil, safflower	Consume much less	
Oil, sesame	Consume much less	
Oil, Shea nut	Consume much less	
Oil, soybean	Consume much less	
Oil, sunflower	Consume much less	
Oil, tea seed	Consume much less	
Oil, tomato seeds	Consume much less	
Oil, Ucuhuba Butter	Consume much less	
Oil, walnut	Consume less	
Oil, wheat germ	More helpful	
Okra	Most helpful	
Olives	Neutral/OK	
Omega-3 fatty acids	Helpful	
Onion rings	Consume much less	
Onions	More helpful; 2-5 oz. of fresh onion daily, or 1 tsp. onion juice 3-4 times a day	
Orange juice	More helpful	
Orange roughy	Helpful	
Oranges	More helpful	
Oregano	Helpful	
Organically grown foods	More helpful	
Ornish Plan & Diet	More helpful	
Oysters	Helpful	
Pancakes	Consume less	
Pancreas (lamb, beef, veal)	Consume less	
Papaya	More helpful	
Parsley	More helpful	
Parsnips	More helpful	
Passion fruit	Most helpful	
Pasta	Neutral/OK	
Pastrami, cured beef	Avoid	
Pastrami, turkey	Avoid	
Peaches	More helpful	
Peaches, dried	Most helpful	
Peanut butter	Helpful	
Peanuts	More helpful	
Pears	More helpful	
Pears, dried	Most helpful	
Peas, green	More helpful	
Peas, split	Most helpful	
Peas, sugar or snap	More helpful	
Pecans	More helpful	

Food Item or Other	Suitability for HBP	Remarks (if any)
Pepper (black or white)	Helpful	
Pepper, banana	More helpful	
Peppermint	Most helpful	
Pepperoni	Avoid	
Peppers, ancho	Most helpful	
Peppers, hot chili	More helpful	
Peppers, hot chili, red	More helpful	
Peppers, jalapeno	More helpful	
Peppers, pasilla	Most helpful	
Peppers, pimento	More helpful	
Perch	More helpful	
Persimmons	More helpful	
Pheasant	Neutral/OK	
Pheasant breast	Neutral/OK	
Phosphorus	Helpful	
Pickle (cucumber)	Consume less	
Pickle relish	Consume less	
Pickle, sweet	Neutral/OK	
Pie crust	Avoid	
Pie, apple	Consume much less	
Pie, coconut cream	Consume much less	
Pie, fried pies (fruit)	Consume much less	
Pie, lemon meringue	Consume less	
Pie, pecan	Consume much less	
Pie, pumpkin	Consume less	
Pie, vanilla cream	Consume much less	
Pigeon peas	Most helpful	
Pike, northern	More helpful	
Pike, walleye	More helpful	
Pili nuts	Most helpful	
Piña colada	Neutral/OK	
Pine nuts	Most helpful	
Pineapple	More helpful	
Pineapple juice	More helpful	
Pistachio nuts	Most helpful	
Pitanga	More helpful	
Pizza	Consume much less	
Plantains	More helpful	
Plum	More helpful	
Pokeberry shoots	More helpful	
Pollock	More helpful	
Pomegranate	More helpful	
Pomegranate juice	More helpful	
Pompano fish	More helpful	
Popcorn, air popped	Most helpful	
Popcorn, oil popped	Consume less	
Poppy seed	Helpful	
Pork back ribs	Consume less	
Pork breakfast strips	Avoid	
Pork cured/ham	Consume much less	
Pork headcheese	Consume much less	

Food Item or Other	Suitability for HBP	Remarks (if any)
Pork heart	Neutral/OK	
Pork kidneys	Neutral/OK	
Pork leg/ham	Neutral/OK	
Pork liver	Neutral/OK	
Pork liver cheese	Avoid	
Pork loin/sirloin	Helpful	
Pork lungs	Neutral/OK	
Pork ribs	Consume less	
Pork shldr	Consume less	
Pork skins	Avoid	
Pork spare ribs	Consume less	
Pork spleen	Neutral/OK	
Potassium	More helpful	
Potato	More helpful	
Potato chips/fried snacks	Helpful	
Potato pancakes	Consume less	
Potato salad	Consume less	
Potato sticks	Consume much less	
Potatoes w/skin	Most helpful	
Pout	More helpful	
Pray, practice your religion	More helpful	
Pretzels	Avoid	
Processed or Refined foods	Consume less	
Protein	Neutral/OK	
Prune juice	Most helpful	
Prunes (dried)	Most helpful	
Pudding	Consume much less	
Puff pastry	Avoid	
Pumelo (Shaddock)	More helpful	
Pumpkin	More helpful	
Pumpkin flowers	More helpful	
Pumpkinseed sunfish	More helpful	
Purslane	More helpful	
Quail	Consume less	
Quail breast	Neutral/OK	
Quince	More helpful	
Quinoa seed	More helpful	
Rabbit meat	Helpful	
Radishes	More helpful	
Raisins	Most helpful	
Raspberries	More helpful	
Raspberries, black	More helpful	
Rhubarb	Helpful	
Rice bran	Most helpful	
Rice cakes (Brown rice based)	Helpful	
Rice, brown	More helpful	
Rice, white	Helpful	
Rice, wild	More helpful	
Rockfish	Helpful	
Rolls, dinner, Kaiser	Consume much less	
Rolls, dinner, whole-wheat	More helpful	

Food Item or Other	Suitability for HBP	Remarks (if any)
Rolls, French	Consume much less	
Rolls, hamburger & hot dog	Consume less	
Rosemary (fresh)	Most helpful	
Rowal	More helpful	
Rutabaga	More helpful	
Rye	Most helpful	
Sablefish	Helpful	
Saffron	Helpful	
Sage	Helpful	
Salad dressing, blue/Roquefort	Avoid	
Salad dressing, French	Avoid	
Salad dressing, Italian	Avoid	
Salami, various	Avoid	
Salmon (smoked, Lox)	Consume much less	
Salmon, pink	Most helpful	
Salt, table	Avoid	
Salted foods, nuts, etc.	Consume much less	
Salt-free or low-salt foods	More helpful	
Sardines	Most helpful	
Sauce, barbecue	Consume much less	
Sauce, cheese	Consume much less	
Sauce, fish	Consume much less	
Sauce, Hoisin	Avoid	
Sauce, oyster	Avoid	
Sauce, pepper or hot	Neutral/OK	
Sauce, Sofrito	Avoid	
Sauce, tabasco	Consume much less	
Sauce, teriyaki	Consume less	
Sauerkraut	Consume less	
Sausage, blood	Avoid	
Sausage, liver	Avoid	
Sausage, meatless	Consume much less	
Sausage, various	Avoid	
Scallops	Helpful	
Scup	More helpful	
Seatrout	Helpful	
Seeds, breadnut tree	Most helpful	
Seeds, chia	Most helpful	
Seeds, cottonseed	Most helpful	
Seeds, flaxseed	Most helpful	
Seeds, pumpkin & squash	Most helpful	
Seeds, safflower	Most helpful	
Seeds, sesame	More helpful	
Seeds, sunflower	Most helpful	
Seeds, watermelon	Most helpful	
Semolina	Helpful	
Sesbania Flower	More helpful	
Shad	More helpful	
Shallots	More helpful	
Shark	More helpful	
Sheepshead	More helpful	

Food Item or Other	Suitability for HBP	Remarks (if any)
Sherbet	Consume less	
Shrimp	Consume less	
Shrimp, breaded	Consume much less	
Sleep 6-8 hours regularly	More helpful	
Smelt	More helpful	
Smoking, tobacco	Consume much less	
Snail	Most helpful	
Snapper	Most helpful	
Sodium (salt)	Consume much less	use spices instead
Soft (carbonated) drinks	Consume less	
Sorghum	Most helpful	
Sound Therapy	Helpful	
Soup, beef broth	Consume less	
Soup, beef stock	Neutral/OK	
Soup, chicken broth	Consume less	
Soup, chicken noodle	Consume less	
Soup, chicken stock	Neutral/OK	
Soup, clam chowder	Neutral/OK	
Soup, fish stock	Helpful	
Soup, minestrone	Neutral/OK	
Soup, veg/beef	Consume less	
Soup, vegetable	Consume less	
Sour cream	Consume less	
Soy milk	Most helpful	
Soy sauce	Consume much less	
Soybean seeds	Most helpful	
Soybeans (green)	Most helpful	
Spaghetti	Neutral/OK	
Spaghetti, spinach	Helpful	
Spaghetti, whole-wheat	Most helpful	
Spearmint (fresh)	More helpful	
Spelt (cooked)	More helpful	
Spinach	More helpful	
Sports drinks	Helpful	
Spot	More helpful	
Squab (pigeon)	Consume less	
Squash, winter	More helpful	
Squash, yellow	More helpful	
Strawberries	More helpful	
Stress	Consume much less	
Sturgeon	More helpful	
Succotash	Helpful	
Sucker	More helpful	
Sugar, brown	Neutral/OK	
Sugar, maple	Helpful	
Sugar, refined	Consume less	
Sugar, table (white or powder)	Consume much less	
Surimi	Helpful	
Sweet potatoes	Helpful	
Sweet potatoes leaves	Most helpful	
Sweet rolls	Consume much less	

Food Item or Other	Suitability for HBP	Remarks (if any)
Swiss chard	Helpful	
Swordfish	Most helpful	
Syrup, chocolate	Consume much less	
Syrup, malt	Consume less	
Syrup, maple	Consume less	
Syrup, sorghum	More helpful	
Syrup, table blends	Consume less	
Taco shells	Consume less	
Tai Chi	More helpful	
Tamarind	Most helpful	
Tangerines	More helpful	
Tapioca	Consume less	
Taro	Most helpful	
Taro chips	Consume less	
Taro leaves	Most helpful	
Taro, Tahitian	Most helpful	
Tarragon (dried)	Helpful	
Tea, green	Consume less	
Tea, herbal	Neutral/OK	
Tea, plain	Consume less	
Tempeh	More helpful	
Thyme (fresh)	Most helpful	
Tilapia	More helpful	
Tilefish	More helpful	
Toasted bread	Helpful	
Tofu	Most helpful	
Tofu, fried	Most helpful	
Tomato juice	Helpful	
Tomato paste	Helpful	
Tomatoes	More helpful	
Tomatoes, sun-dried	Most helpful	
Tonic water	Helpful	
Tortilla chips	Neutral/OK	
Tortillas (corn)	Helpful	
Triticale	Most helpful	
Trout	Most helpful	
Tuna, blue fin	Most helpful	
Tuna, canned	Helpful	
Tuna, yellowfin	More helpful	
Turbot	Helpful	
Turkey breast	Helpful	
Turkey dark meat	Helpful	
Turkey giblets	Consume less	
Turkey heart	Consume less	
Turkey liver	Neutral/OK	
Turkey skins	Consume much less	
Turmeric	Helpful	
Turnip greens	Most helpful	
Turnips	More helpful	
Veal heart	Consume less	
Veal kidneys	Helpful	

Food Item or Other	Suitability for HBP	Remarks (if any)
Veal liver	Helpful	
Veal loin	Neutral/OK	
Veal lungs	Neutral/OK	
Veal shank	Helpful	
Veal shoulder/leg/sirloin	Neutral/OK	
Veal spleen	Neutral/OK	
Veal thymus	Helpful	
Veal tongue	Consume less	
Vegetable shortening	Consume much less	
Vegetarian diet	Helpful	
Venison	Helpful	
Vine spinach (Basella)	Most helpful	
Vinegar	Neutral/OK	
Vitamin D	Helpful	
Waffles	Consume less	
Walk, wheel, or jog	More helpful	
Walnuts	Most helpful	
Walnuts, black	Most helpful	
Wasabi root	Most helpful	
Water	Helpful	
Watercress	More helpful	
Watermelon	More helpful	
Wheat	Helpful	
Wheat bran	Most helpful	
Wheat germ	Most helpful	
Whelk	Most helpful	
Whey (dried)	Most helpful	
Whiskey	Neutral/OK	
White fish	Most helpful	
White fish (smoked)	Helpful	
Whiting	More helpful	
Whole-wheat	Most helpful	
Wild fish and free range animals	Helpful	
Wine, red	Helpful	
Wine, white	Helpful	
Winged beans leaves	More helpful	
Wolffish	More helpful	
Yam	Most helpful	
Yellowtail	More helpful	
Yoga	More helpful	certain postures must be avoided
Yogurt	Neutral/OK	
Yucca	More helpful	
Zucchini	More helpful	

High Cholesterol (& HBP)

Cholesterol is a fat-like substance found in every cell of your body. Your body needs cholesterol to function properly, and it normally produces the amount of cholesterol that it requires. However, many foods that you consume can also result in increase in the level of cholesterol in your body -- in your blood in particular. There is usually no symptom for high cholesterol, but it can be discovered through a routine blood test.

High levels of cholesterol in your blood can result in build-up of what is known as plaque in your arteries. Plaque can narrow or block your arteries. Since arteries carry blood from your heart to the rest of your body, high level of cholesterol can result in heart disease and damage your cardiovascular system.

Cholesterol exists in two forms in your blood known as: LDL and HDL. LDL is called bad cholesterol because it leads to build up of plaque in your arteries. HDL is called good cholesterol because it removes and carries cholesterol away and delivers it to your liver where it gets eliminated from your body.

Your LDL is considered too high if it is greater than 160 milligram per deciliter. Your HDL is considered too low if it is less than 40 mg/dl. Your total cholesterol is considered too high if it is greater than 240 mg/dl, and is considered desirable if it is less than 200 mg/dl.

You are likely to have high cholesterol if you consume too much animal fat and trans fatty acids, you are not physically active, you are overweight, and there is a history of the same in your family. Your cholesterol levels tend to rise as you get older.

__Choose__ these for High Cholesterol & High Blood Pressure

Top 5 items to choose:

Garlic; Whole grains; Dried Fruits; Seeds; Soymilk;

Food items and actions that could improve your health (within a food group, most helpful items are listed first):

Meat, Fish & Poultry

Marlin; Swordfish; White fish; Trout; Snapper; Sardines; Blue fin tuna; Ling; Sturgeon; Carp; Spot; Monkfish; Tilefish; Pollock; Seabass; Halibut; Freshwater bass; Bluefish; King mackerel; Pink salmon; Whiting; Striped bass; Yellowfin tuna; Smelt; Yellowtail; Drum; Sucker; Wolffish; Fish roe; Cisco (smoked); Scup; Pout; Milkfish; Shark; Catfish; Mackerel; Cusk; Tilapia; Pike; Surimi; Shad; Herring; Mullet; Lingcod; Pompano fish; Sheepshead; Cisco; Rockfish; Perch; Flatfish (flounder & sole); Canned tuna; Butterfish; Mussels; Grouper; Sablefish; Anchovy; Seatrout; Dolphinfish (Mahi-Mahi); Pumpkinseed sunfish; White fish (smoked); Turbot; Burbot; Haddock; Caviar; Snail; Cod; Croaker; Chicken breast (no skin); Orange roughy; Octopus; Whelk; Scallops; Spiny lobster; Dungeness crab; Clams; Pheasant; Oysters; Veal loin; Beef filet mignon;

Eggs, Beans, Nuts and Seeds

Split peas; Seeds: breadnut tree, chia, sunflower; Soy milk; Beans: adzuki, navy; Soybeans (green); various beans; Chickpeas; Lentils; Ginkgo nuts; Black walnuts; Pistachio nuts; Black-eyed peas; Soybean seeds; Hazelnuts or Filberts; Safflower seeds; Lupin; Sugar or snap peas; Breadfruit seeds; Walnuts; Pine nuts; Green peas; Almonds (sweet in particular); Flaxseed; Beechnuts; Butternuts; Sesame seeds; Peanuts; Pumpkin & squash seeds; Acorns; Alfalfa sprouts; Cornnuts; Chestnuts; Hickory nuts; Cottonseed; Brazil nuts; Pecans; Watermelon seeds; Cashew nuts; Pili nuts; Egg white;

Fruits & Juices

Dried fruits especially: Banana, Litchi, Prunes, Figs, Peaches, Raisins, Apricots & Currants; Tamarind; Goji berry; Dates; Passion fruit; Abiyuch; Elderberries; Guava; Currants (raw); Kiwi fruit; Avocado; Blackberries; various berries; Cantaloupe; Kumquats; Rowal; Apricots; Lemon; Banana; Cranberry juice; Breadfruit; Pineapple juice; Grapefruit; Plum; Lime; Jujube (fruit); Longans; Mango; Persimmons; Peaches; Plantains; Prune juice; Pumelo (Shaddock); Durian; Papaya; Grapes; Grape juice; Grapefruit juice; Figs; Pomegranate; Natal Plum (Carissa); Acerola; Litchi; Pineapple; Cherries; Watermelon; Tangerines; Nectarine; Strawberries; Rhubarb; Pomegranate juice; Pitanga; Cranberries; Olives; Honeydew melon; Quince; Pears; Apples (eat with skin); Blueberries and Bilberries; Oranges; Apple juice (use fresh apples w/skin); Orange juice;

Vegetables

Garlic; Fungi cloud ears; Grape leaves; Shitake mushrooms; Peppers: ancho, pasilla; Pigeon peas; Sun-dried tomatoes; Wasabi root; Taro leaves; Corn bran; Sweet potatoes leaves; Dandelion Greens; Garden cress; Kale; Chrysanthemum (Garland); Mustard spinach; Balsam pear leafy tips; Amaranth leaves; Chinese broccoli; Chicory greens; Collards; Mustard greens; Turnip greens; Taro; Vine spinach (Basella); Bok choy; Watercress; Arugula; Beet greens; Balsam pear; Broccoli; Brussels sprouts; Endive; Kohlrabi; Carrots; Okra; Winged beans leaves; Spinach; Epazote; Savoy cabbage; Jalapeno peppers; Cauliflower; Banana peppers; Chrysanthemum Leaves; Green onions (scallions); Red cabbage; various peppers; Pokeberry shoots; Arrowhead; Green cabbage; Portabella mushrooms; Lotus root; Parsnips; Yam; Borage; Cowpeas leafy tips; Swiss chard; Onions (2-5 oz. of fresh onion daily, or 1 tsp. onion juice 3-4 times a day); Quinoa seed; Winter squash; Nopal; Potatoes w/skin; Romaine & Loose leaf lettuce; Pumpkin; Purslane; Sesbania Flower; Tomatoes; Fiddlehead ferns; Green beans; Shallots; Kelp; Artichoke; Rutabaga; Sweet potatoes; Arrowroot; Asparagus; Corn; Tomato juice; Celtuce; Yellow squash; Zucchini; Jew's ear mushrooms; Pumpkin flowers; Radishes; Lambsquarters; Potato; other vegetables;

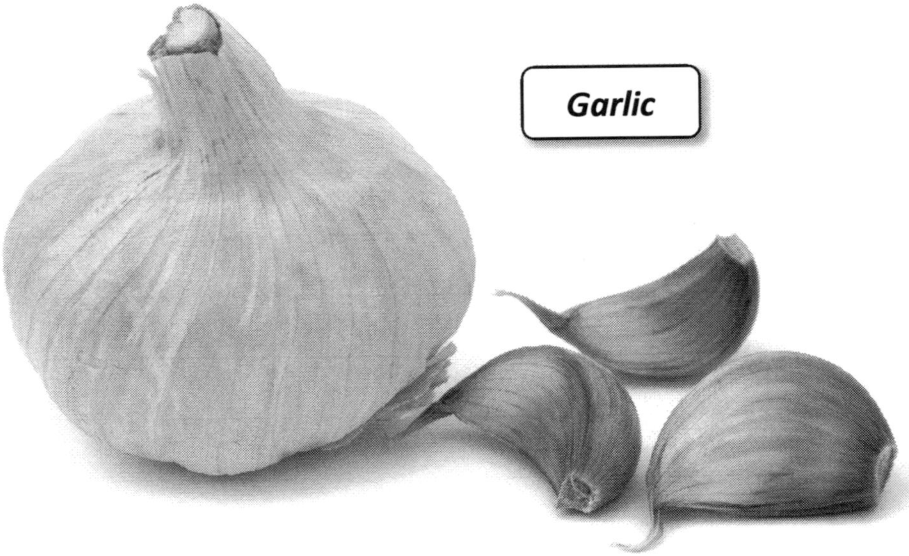

Garlic

Breads, Grains, Cereals, Pasta

Wheat germ; Whole-wheat; Whole-wheat bread; Durum wheat; Rye; Whole-wheat English muffins; Whole-wheat cereal; Wheat germ cereal; Bran flakes cereal; Sorghum; Wheat bran cereal; Whole-wheat spaghetti; Barley; Rice bran; Triticale; Oatmeal (cereal); Wheat germ bread; Spelt (cooked); Wheat bran; Amaranth; Buckwheat; Oats; Bulgur; Whole-wheat dinner rolls; Millet; Brown rice; Whole-wheat crackers; Rice cakes (Brown rice based); Wild rice; Shredded wheat cereal; Oat bran (3 grams daily); Oat bran muffins; Oat bran bread; Tortillas (corn); Granola cereal; Pumpernickel bread; Semolina; Chinese chow Mein noodles; Italian bread; Corn flakes; Bread sticks; Corn muffins;

Dairy Products, Fats & Oils

Wheat Germ Oil; Whey (dried); Flaxseed Oil; Yogurt; Salmon fish oil; Cottage Cheese; Cod liver fish oil; Fat-free or low fat Dairy Products; Salt-free or low-salt Dairy Products

Desserts, Snacks, Beverages

Air-popped Popcorn; Sesame crunch candies; Peanut butter; Molasses; Water; Red wine; Oil popped popcorn; Potato chips/fried snacks; Peanut bar candy; White wine;

Herbs & Spices, Prepared & Fast Foods

Thyme (fresh); Whole-grain Cornmeal; Tofu; Tempeh; Peppermint; Parsley; Rosemary (fresh); Natto; Tomato paste; Mustard seed; Coriander/Cilantro; Miso; Cottonseed meal; Dill weed; Turmeric; Mace; Poppy seed; French fries; Spearmint (fresh); Cocoa; Cheese fondue; Ginger; Basil (fresh); Sage; Tarragon (dried); Egg rolls (veg); Succotash; Oregano; Malt syrup; Croutons; Cayenne (red) pepper; Cinnamon; Clam chowder; Sorghum syrup; Fennel seeds; Saffron; Pepper (black or white); Cloves; Fish stock; Corn cakes; Corn salad;

Alternative Therapies & Miscellaneous

Consult your doctor; Exercise; Fat-free or low fat products; Follow DASH diet; Ornish Plan & Diet; Fresh (uncooked) fruits/veg's or use no salt added canned; 1-2 alcoholic drinks/day; Glucomannan; Meditation; Pray, practice your religion; Sleep 6-8 hours regularly; Tai Chi; Vegetarian diet; Yoga (certain postures must be avoided); Salt-free or low-salt foods; Organically grown foods;

Key Nutrients & Herbal Medicines

Celery seed; Fiber; Yucca; Hawthorn (in berries form or tea from dried leaves and flowers. Do not take with other heart medications); Omega-3 fatty acids; Psyllium; Fenugreek seeds; Calcium; Monounsaturated fat (limit to 20% of total daily calories); Siberian Ginseng; Magnesium; Potassium; Vitamin B-3 (Niacin; in Nicotinic acid form);

<u>Do not</u> choose these for High Cholesterol & High Blood Pressure

Top 5 items to avoid:

Luncheon (Processed) meats; Hydrogenated vegetable oil; Sweets; Butter & Margarine; Animal fat & Lard;

Avoid or consume much less of the following (within a food group, most harmful items are listed first):

Meat, Fish & Poultry

Chorizo; Pepperoni; Sausages; Frankfurters; Luncheon meats; Beerwurst beer salami; Pork skins; Pork liver cheese; Pastramis; Cured beef; Bologna; Beef jerky sticks; Salamis; Pork breakfast strips; Cured meats; Beef chuck/brisket; Beef/Lamb tongue; Bacon; Pork ribs; Chicken & Turkey skins; Chicken heart; Pork spare ribs; Organ meats; Beef ribs; Squab (pigeon); Lamb ribs; Corned beef; Beef; Pork; Ground lamb; Goose; Lamb; Bison/buffalo meat; Chicken dark meat; Shrimp; Turkey dark meat; Meatless sausage; Lobster;

Instead <u>choose</u>: Chicken liver; Alaskan King crab; Beef liver; Eel; Salmon (smoked, Lox); Quail breast; Crayfish; Blue crab; Guinea hen; Pork loin/sirloin; Cuttlefish; Veal shank; Abalone; Turkey breast; Calamari; Veal shoulder/leg/sirloin; Rabbit meat; Quail;

Eggs, Beans, Nuts and Seeds

Coconut milk; Egg substitute; Egg; Coconut; Egg yolk; Coconut meat (dried)

Instead <u>choose</u>: Macadamia Nuts

Breads, Grains, Cereals, Pasta

Croissant; Danish pastry; Sweet cinnamon rolls; Saltines crackers; Donuts; Milk crackers; Kaiser dinner rolls; Wheat crackers; French rolls; Waffles; Hamburger & hot dog rolls; Cream of wheat; Matzo crackers; White bread;

Instead <u>choose</u>: Spinach spaghetti; Wheat; English muffins; White rice; Banana bread; Egg noodles; Japanese noodles; Rice noodles; Spaghetti; Cornbread; Biscuits;

Dairy Products, Fats & Oils

Hydrogenated vegetable oil; Margarine-like spreads; Butter (salted); Animal fat; Ucuhuba Butter oil; Brie cheese; Lard; Vegetable shortening; Margarine; Poultry fat; Babassu oil; Cheese: Roquefort, goat, pimento; Cupu Assu oil; Feta cheese; Butter (unsalted); various cheese; various seeds/nuts/vegetable oils; Whipped cream; Cream; Sour cream; Chocolate milk; Non-dairy creamers; Skim milk;

Instead <u>choose:</u> Herring fish oil; Oils: canola, walnut, olive; Menhaden fish oil; Sardine fish oil; 2% fat milk;

Desserts, Snacks, Beverages

Pound cake; Butter cookies; Chocolate cake; Sweet chocolate; Éclairs; Puff pastry; various cakes; Cream puffs; Dessert toppings; Chocolate mousse; Cheesecake; various cookies; Chocolate ice cream; After-dinner mints; Vanilla cream pie; Vanilla ice cream; Carob candies; Pudding; Pie crust; various pies; Chocolate (use cocoa powder or carob instead); Fruit leather/rolls; Coffeecake; Pretzels; Coffee liqueur; Potato sticks; Coffee; Chewing gum; Jams & Preserves; Sherbet; Candies; Pancakes; Taro chips; Fruit punch; Lemonade; Frostings; Soft (carbonated) drinks; Eggnog; Honey; Frozen yogurt;

Instead <u>choose</u>: Green tea (do not brew or drink tea scolding hot); Tonic water; Halvah; Tortilla chips; Plain tea; Beer; Sports drinks; Applesauce; Crème de menthe; Ginger ale; Piña colada; Herbal tea; Pumpkin pie;

Herbs & Spices. Prepared & Fast Foods

Foie gras or liver pate; Blue/Roquefort salad dressing; Hot dog; Cheese sauce; Nachos; French salad dressing; Pizza; Chocolate syrup; Oyster sauce; Chicken Nuggets; Italian salad dressing; Breaded shrimp; various sauces; Table sugar (white or powder); Table salt; Tabasco sauce; Ketchup; Cheeseburger; Soy sauce; Capers; Macaroni; Tapioca; Hush puppies; Mayonnaise; Onion rings; French toast; Potato salad; Syrup (table blends); Maple syrup; Hamburger; Potato pancakes; Pickle (cucumber); Gravies (canned); Beef broth; Chicken broth; Chicken noodle soup;

Instead <u>choose</u>: Minestrone soup; Falafel; Horseradish; Chervil; Hummus; Cole slaw; Cardamom; Vegetable soup; Chives; Tortilla chips; Teriyaki sauce; Sweet pickle; Nutmeg; Sauerkraut; Veg/beef soup; Couscous; Brown sugar; Vinegar;

Alternative Therapies & Miscellaneous

2+ alcoholic drinks/day; Excess body weight; Smoking, tobacco; Processed or Refined foods; Fried or battered foods; Baking using butter; Hyperthermia (avoid if extremely high blood pressure); Stress; Salted foods, nuts, etc.; Canned foods; Corn sweetener; Sugared fruit juice or from concentrate;

Key Nutrients & Herbal Medicines

Saturated fat (limit to 7% of daily calories); Cholesterol (less than 200 mg per day); Caffeine; Total fat (limit to 25-35% of total daily calories); Licorice; Sodium (salt); Trans fatty acids;

High Triglycerides (& HBP)

Triglycerides are a type of fat that exist in the bloodstream, in fat tissues and in foods. Triglycerides can be produced from fats in the foods we consume, from carbohydrates, or from calories not used by the tissues immediately after consumption and stored in the fat cells for future use.

High level of triglycerides in the blood can result in hardening and narrowing of arteries, leading to greater possibility of heart attack and strokes. This condition often occurs along with high level of cholesterol in the blood stream. It is often discovered in the same blood test that measures cholesterol level. Triglycerides level is considered high if it is greater than 200 milligrams per deci-liter.

The most likely causes for having high triglycerides are:

- drinking too much alcohol,
- being overweight,
- consuming too much sugars and carbohydrates
- suffering from other medical conditions such as diabetes or kidney failure

Proper nutrition and exercise can be very effective in lowering the triglycerides level in your blood.

Choose these for High Triglycerides & High Blood Pressure

Top 5 items to choose:

Fish; Fish Roe; Flaxseed & Chia seeds; Soy milk/Soybeans; Garlic;

Food items and actions that could improve your health (within a food group, most helpful items are listed first):

Meat, Fish & Poultry

Salmon; Swordfish; Trout; White fish; Blue fin tuna; Fish roe; Sardines; Ling; Mackerel; Spot; Herring; Sturgeon; Tilefish; Bluefish; Monkfish; Marlin; Yellowtail; Shad; Milkfish; Seabass; Smoked cisco; Scup; Smelt; Pollock; Shark; Various bass; Yellowfin tuna; Carp; Pout; Halibut; Whiting; Wolffish; Caviar; Mussels; Sucker; Snapper; Drum; Mullet; Anchovy; Pike; Pompano fish; Canned tuna; Snail; Spiny lobster; Smoked salmon (lox); Sablefish; Surimi; Perch; Catfish; Mahi-mahi; Portabella mushrooms; Tilapia; Octopus; Lingcod; Cusk; Cisco; Grouper; Skinless chicken breast; Whelk; Fried calamari; Rockfish; Sheepshead; Butterfish; Flatfish; Burbot; Seatrout; Oysters; Millet; Turbot; Haddock; Veal shank; Veal loin; Eel; Scallops; Cod; Crayfish; Pork loin/sirloin; Beef filet mignon; Quail breast; Clams; Blue crab; Pheasant; Smoked whitefish; Abalone; Turkey breast; Orange roughy; Guinea hen; Venison; Cuttlefish; Veal shoulder/leg/sirloin;

Eggs, Beans, Nuts and Seeds

Flaxseeds; Soy milk; Chia seeds; Soybean seeds; Soybeans (green); Walnuts; Sunflower seeds; Ginkgo nuts; Breadfruit seeds; Safflower seeds; Peanuts; Almonds; Pine nuts; Split peas; various beans; Lentils; Breadnut tree seeds; Hazelnuts; Butternuts; Chickpeas; Alfalfa sprouts; Green peas; Cottonseeds; Sugar or snap peas; Pumpkin & squash seeds; Lupin; Watermelon seeds; Black-eyed peas; Pistachio nuts; Beechnuts; Sesame seeds; Chestnuts;

Fruits & Juices

Passion fruit; Avocado; Dried Peaches; Berries; Guava; Currants; Kiwi fruit; Prunes; Lemon; Lime; Dried apricots; Apricots; Cantaloupe; Jujube; Banana; Tamarind; Pitanga; Pumelo; Strawberries; Dates; Persimmons; Pears; Dried banana; Kumquats; Peaches; Breadfruit; Blueberries and Bilberries; Grapefruit; Honeydew melon; Nectarine; Oranges; Papaya; Pineapple; Plum; Watermelon; Dried figs; Apples; Plantains; Mango; Tangerines; Raisins; Pomegranate;

Vegetables

Shitake mushrooms; Garlic; Ancho & Pasilla peppers; Sun-dried tomatoes; Fungi Cloud Ears; Artichoke; Taro leaves; Onions (2-5 oz. of fresh onion daily, or 1 tsp. onion juice 3-4 times a day); Hot chili peppers; Pigeon peas; Grape leaves; Sweet potato leaves; Wasabi Root; Arrowhead; Kelp; Chicory greens; Dandelion Greens; Mustard spinach; Garden cress; Kale; Corn bran; Arugula; Nopal; Collards; Mustard greens; Okra; Turnip greens; Potatoes w/skin; Cauliflower; Broccoli; Endive; Bok choy; Borage; Purslane; Watercress; Hot peppers; Yam; Parsnips; Beet greens; Brussels sprouts; Carrots; Green onions (scallions); Kohlrabi; Jew's ear mushroom; Quinoa seed; Corn; Lotus root; Celtuce; Rutabaga; Spinach; Squash; Zucchini; ... other vegetables.

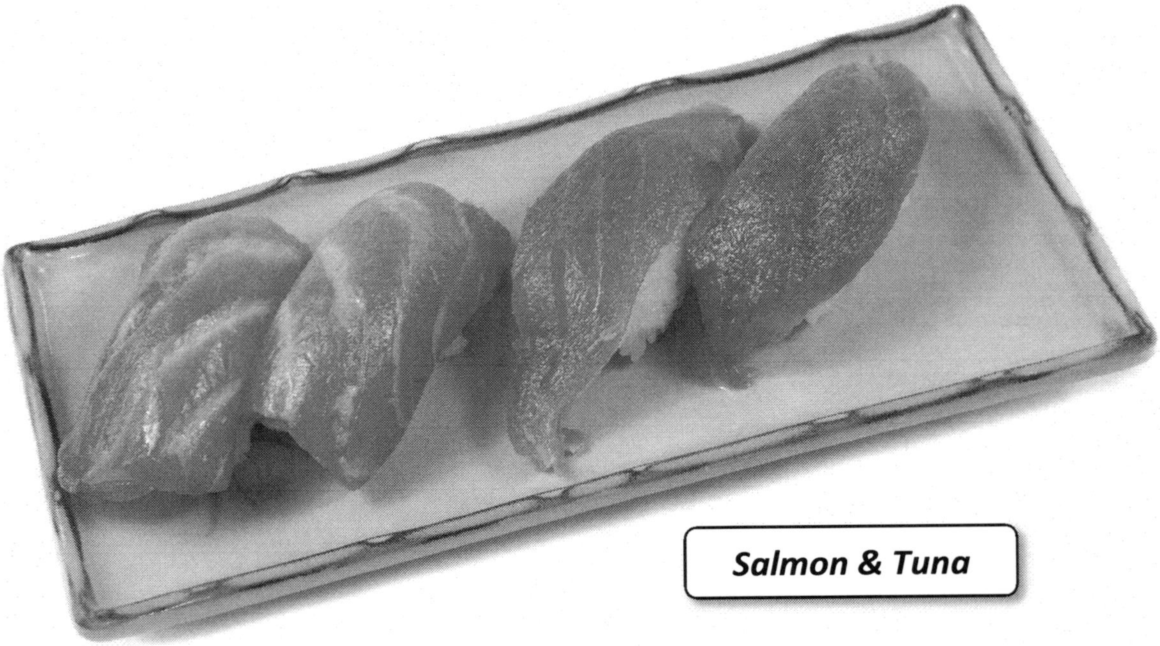

Breads, Grains, Cereals, Pasta

Wheat bran; Wheat germ; Rice bran; Buckwheat; Durum wheat; Whole-wheat cereal; Whole-wheat bread; Wheat germ cereal; Whole-wheat; Whole-wheat English muffins; Bran flakes cereal; Whole-wheat Spaghetti; Rye; Wheat germ bread; Amaranth; Oats; Triticale; Oatmeal; Rice cakes; Wheat Bran muffins; Spelt; Sorghum; Millet; Brown rice; Shredded wheat; Barley; Bulgur; Whole-wheat dinner rolls; Wild rice; Oat bran muffins; Oat bran bread; Tortillas (corn); Whole-wheat crackers;

Dairy Products, Fats & Oils

Wheat germ oil; Fish Oil: Cod Liver, Sardine; Flaxseed Oil; Fish Oils: Herring, Menhaden, Salmon; Dried whey; Cottage cheese; Fat-free or Low Fat Dairy products

Desserts, Snacks, Beverages

Soy Milk; Air Popped Popcorn; Grape Juice; Orange Juice; Cranberry juice; Apple Juice; Grapefruit Juice; Peanut butter; Pomegranate juice; Water; Tomato juice; ***Avoid fruit juices made from concentrate or with added sugar***

Herbs & Spices, Fast Foods, Prepared Foods

Tofu; Tempeh; Cottonseed Meal; Thyme; Peppermint; Whole-grain Corn Meal; Natto; Ginger; Miso; Rosemary; Dill Weed; Cinnamon; Parsley; Red or cayenne pepper; Spearmint; Tarragon; Teriyaki sauce; Coriander/Cilantro; Basil; French fries; Succotash; Soup, fish stock; Oregano; Sage; Tomato paste;

Alternative Therapies & Miscellaneous

Exercise (including cardiovascular, weight training, Tai chi and Yoga); Follow DASH diet; Fresh (uncooked) Fruits/vegetables; Meditation; Pray, Practice your religion; Sleep, Rest 6-8 hours regularly; Follow Ornish plan & diet; Salt-free or low-salt foods; Organically grown foods; Wild fish and free range animals;

Key Nutrients & Herbal Meds

Omega-3 Fatty Acids; Hawthorn (in berries form or tea from dried leaves and flowers); Calcium; Celery seeds; Siberian ginseng; Magnesium; Potassium; Vitamin B-3 (Niacin; in Nicotinic acid form); Yucca;

<u>Do not</u> choose these for High Triglycerides & High Blood Pressure

Top 5 items to avoid:

Sugar/Sweets; Margarine; Hydrogenated Vegetable Oil; Luncheon (processed) Meats; Butter; & Excess Body Weight

Avoid or consume much less of the following (within a food group, most harmful items are listed first):

Meat, Fish & Poultry

Pepperoni; various Sausage; Frankfurters; Luncheon (processed) Meats; various Salami; Chorizo; Beef jerky sticks; various Bologna; Pork skin; various Pastrami; Tongue (Beef, veal, lamb); Poultry skin; Cured Meats; Bacon; Beef chuck/brisket; Organ meats; Corned Beef; Pork ribs; Beef; Lamb ribs; Pork; Lamb; Goose; Liver; Meatless sausage;

Instead <u>choose</u>: Rabbit meat; Duck; Croaker; Quail; Turkey dark meat; Lobster; Beef round steak; Shrimp; Beef rib eye; Boar meat;

Eggs, Beans, Nuts and Seeds

Coconut Milk; Egg Yolk; Coconut; Egg substitute; Egg;

Instead <u>choose</u>: Brazil nuts; Hickory nuts; Cashew nuts; Acorns; Pili nuts; Pecans; Cornnuts; Egg white;

Fruits & Juices

There are no fruits that can worsen your conditions.

Vegetables

There are no vegetables that can worsen your conditions.

Breads, Grains, Cereals, Pasta

Croissant; Danish Pastry; Donuts; Saltines crackers; Sweet Rolls; various Crackers; Granola Bars; Cornbread; Waffles; Kaiser dinner rolls; Biscuits; French rolls; Bagels; Banana bread;

Instead <u>choose</u>: Pumpernickel bread; Semolina; Oat bran; Spinach spaghetti; White rice; Corn flakes; Italian bread; Cream of wheat cereal; Granola cereal;

Dairy Products, Fats & Oils

Margarine; Margarine-Like Spreads; Hydrogenated Vegetable Oil; Butter; various Shortening; Animal Fat; Lard; Brie cheese; Oil Of various Vegetables, Seeds and Nuts; American cheese; Various cheese; Whipped cream; Cream; Whole milk; Sour Cream; Non-Dairy Cream Substitutes; Gruyere cheese; Ricotta cheese; Swiss cheese; Skim milk; Mustard oil; Chocolate Milk; Olive oil;

Instead <u>choose</u>: Walnut oil; Yogurt; Canola oil;

Desserts, Snacks, Beverages

Cakes; Sweet Chocolate; Cookies; Puff Pastry; Éclairs; Cheesecake; Cream Puffs; Dessert Toppings; Pie crust; Chocolate Mousse; various types Of Pies; Fruit Leather/Rolls; After-Dinner Mints; various Ice Cream; Coffee Liqueur; Frostings; Honey; Candies; Chewing Gum; Jams & Preserves; Pudding; Jellies; Sherbet; Ice cream cones; Crème De Menthe; Soft (Carbonated) Drinks; Frozen Yogurt; Sugared or from concentrate fruit juices; Fruit punch; Lemonade; Pancakes; Dark chocolate; Taro Chips; Oil-popped popcorn; Piña Colada; Coffee; 80+ Proof distilled alcoholic beverages; Whiskey; Milk shakes;

Instead choose: Sports drinks; Wine; Ginger ale; Green Tea;

Herbs & Spices, Fast Foods, Prepared Foods

Foie Gras or Liver Pate; Breaded Shrimp; Table Sugar (white or powdered); Blue/Roquefort salad dressing; Chocolate Syrup; Various salad dressing; Onion Rings; Nachos; Various Fast Foods; Hoisin sauce; Pizza; various Syrups; Barbecue sauce; Mayonnaise; Various sauces; Table Salt; Taco Shells; Ketchup; Potato sticks; Pretzels; Capers; Brown Sugar; Hash brown potatoes; Maple Sugar; Tapioca; Tabasco sauce; Pickle relish; Nutmeg; Potato Pancakes; French Toast; Macaroni; Sweet pickle; Potato salad; Mustard; Fish sauce; Pickle; Canned gravies;

Instead choose: Chervil; Poppy seed; Cheese fondue; Clam chowder; Black & white pepper; Turmeric; Mustard seed; Soy sauce; Corn salad; Mints; Saffron;

Alternative Therapies & Miscellaneous

Excess body weight; Over two drinks of alcoholic beverages per day; Smoking. Tobacco; Corn sweetener; Preparing food fried or battered; Hyperthermia; Stress; Salted foods, nuts, etc.; Canned foods; Baking using butter; Sweeteners;

Key Nutrients & Herbal Meds

Saturated fat (limit to 7% of daily calories); Trans fatty acids; Caffeine; Licorice; Sodium/salt (limit to 1,500 mg per day); Refined Sugar;

Gout (& HBP)

Gout is a common and painful condition that affects your joints. It is a form of arthritis and can attack any of your joints but it often attacks joints in your big toe first.

Gout is caused by build-up of uric acid in your blood. When uric acid is stored as crystals in your joints, it creates inflammation, pain and stiffness. Uric acid builds up in your blood if you consume too much of certain foods (foods rich in purines), or if your body produces more uric acid than it eliminates. Too much alcohol consumption can adversely affect body's ability to eliminate uric acid in the blood.

You are most likely to get gout if:

- you have a family history of the disease,
- you are a man,
- you are between 40 and 50 years old,
- you drink too much alcohol,
- you are overweight,
- you consume too much of foods rich in purines (e.g., dry beans, certain fish and animal organs),
- you suffer from other medical conditions (e.g., kidney problems, high blood pressure), or
- you take certain medications (e.g., aspirin, diuretics, Niacin).

__Choose__ these for Gout & High Blood Pressure

Top 5 items to consume:

Whole Grains; Cereals; Goji berries & Currants; Fruit Juices; Tofu;

Food items and actions that could improve your health (within a food group, most helpful items are listed first):

Meat, Fish & Poultry

There are no items in this food group that can improve your health conditions. But there are many items that are neutral for you listed in the next section.

Eggs, Beans, Nuts and Seeds

Soy milk; Breadnut tree seeds; Ginkgo nuts; Chia seeds; Flaxseed; Safflower seeds; Breadfruit seeds; Butternuts; Pine nuts; Pistachio Nuts; Cotton seeds; Chestnuts; Almonds; Hazelnuts or Filberts; Pumpkin & squash seeds; Pili nuts; Beechnuts; Cashew nuts; Walnuts; Acorns; Hickory nuts; Brazil nuts; Cornnuts; Navy beans; Pecans; Sunflower seeds; Soybeans (green); Sugar or snap peas; Chickpeas;

Fruits & Juices

Goji berry; Cranberry juice; Currants; Tamarind; Orange juice; Cherries (especially tart, including juice); Pineapple juice; Guava; Blackberries; Grapefruit juice; Dried Pears; various berries; Jujube; Longans; Persimmons; Dried Peaches; Grape juice; Prune juice; Kumquats; Lemon; Prunes; Breadfruit; Litchi; Apple juice; Passion Fruit; Oranges; Kiwi Fruit; Apples; Grapefruit; Plantains; Papaya; Dried banana; Durian; Lime; Nectarine; Strawberries; Pomegranate juice; Cranberries; Dried fruits; Rhubarb; Mango; Plum; Avocado; Figs; Pomegranate; Peaches; Pineapple; Tangerines; Pears; Watermelon; Banana; Dates; Honeydew Melon; Grapes; Cantaloupe; Apricots; Quince; Raisins; Olives;

Vegetables

Taro leaves; Wasabi Root; Vine spinach (Basella); Sun-dried Tomatoes; Mustard spinach; Garden cress; Dandelion Greens; Quinoa seed; Grape leaves; Peppers: ancho, pasilla; Pigeon peas; Potatoes w/skin; Arrowhead; Balsam pear; Yam; Watercress; Corn bran; Sweet potatoes leaves; Hot peppers; Borage; Arugula; Chicory greens; Okra; Tomato juice; Turnip greens; Beet greens; Pokeberry shoots; Garlic; Kelp; Purslane; Lotus root; Taro; Celery; Onions (2-5 oz. of fresh onion daily, or 1 tsp. onion juice 3-4 times a day); Bell peppers; Bok choy; Parsnips; Kohlrabi; Green onions (scallions); Tomatoes; Kale; Celtuce; Zucchini; Lambsquarters; Pumpkin flowers; Shallots; Arrowroot; Mustard greens; Brussels sprouts; Winter Squash; Swiss chard; Cabbage; Artichoke; Collards; Carrots; Endive; Broccoli; Cucumbers with peel; various lettuce; Beets; Hearts of palm; Radishes; Fungi cloud ears; Shitake mushrooms; Rutabaga; Yellow squash; Sweet potatoes; Fennel; Eggplant; Turnips;

Breads, Grains, Cereals, Pasta

Amaranth; Buckwheat; Bran flakes cereal; Triticale; Sorghum; Durum wheat; Shredded wheat; Wheat germ cereal; Oatmeal; Whole-wheat cereal; Bulgur; Granola cereal; Whole-wheat English Muffins; Spelt; Whole-wheat bread; Rye; Millet; Wild rice; Whole-wheat spaghetti; Brown rice; Various bread; Corn flakes cereal; Cream of wheat; whole-wheat dinner rolls; Rice Bran; Wheat Bran; Oat Bran Muffins; White rice; English muffins; Oats; Wheat Bran Muffins; Barley; Rice crisps; Whole-wheat crackers; Pasta; Spaghetti; Bagels; Rice cakes; Waffles; Wheat germ; Tortillas (corn);

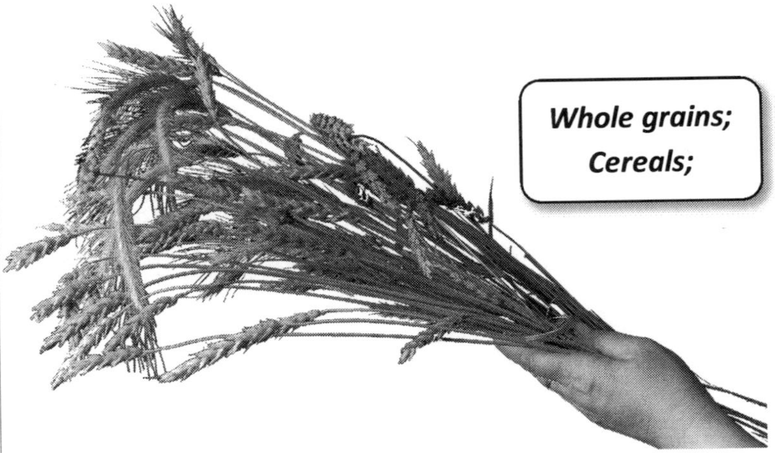

Dairy Products, Fats & Oils

Dried whey; Cottage cheese; Milk; Gjetost cheese; Swiss cheese; Yogurt; Gruyere cheese; Fat-Free or Low Fat Products;

Desserts, Snacks, Beverages

Air-popped Popcorn; Water; Tonic Water; Sports drinks; Ginger Ale; Sesame crunch candies; Milk shakes; Oil popped popcorn; Hot Chocolate; Blackstrap molasses; Wine; ***__Avoid__* fruit juices made from concentrate or sugared**

Herbs & Spices, Fast Foods, Prepared Foods

Whole-grain Cornmeal; Tofu; Thyme; Peppermint; Rosemary; Parsley; French fries; Dill Weed; Natto; Cheese Fondue; Spearmint; coriander/cilantro; Basil; tarragon; Egg rolls; sage; Corn salad; Potato pancakes; Succotash; Taco shells; Oregano; Fennel seeds;

Alternative Therapies & Miscellaneous

Exercise; Fluids/juices/water; Follow DASH diet; Fresh/uncooked fruits & vegetables; Meditation; Ornish Plan & Diet; Pray. Practice your religion; Sleep. Rest 6-8 hours regularly; Tai Chi; Yoga (certain postures must be avoided); Salt-free or low-salt foods; Organically grown foods;

Key Nutrients & Herbal Meds

Celery seed; Hawthorn (in berries form or tea from dried leaves and flowers; do not take with other heart medications); Fenugreek; Calcium; Siberian Ginseng; Magnesium; Potassium; Starch/complex carbohydrates; Yucca;

<u>Do not</u> choose these for Gout & High Blood Pressure

Top 5 items to avoid:

Excess body weight; Chocolate; Bacon/Cured & Processed Meats; 2+ alcoholic drinks/day; Margarine & Hydrogenated vegetable oil;

Avoid or consume much less of the following (within a food group, most harmful items are listed first):

Meat, Fish & Poultry

Cured Meats; Chorizo; Frankfurters; Luncheon (processed) Meats; Pepperoni; various Sausage; various Salami; Bacon; Pork skin; Pastrami (including turkey); various Bologna; Poultry skin; Corned Beef; Pork cured/ham; Beef chuck/brisket; Tongue (beef, veal, lamb); Squab (pigeon); Pork; Lamb ribs; Beef; Goose; Liver; Quail; Bison/Buffalo Meat; Dark Meat Chicken w/skin; Organ Meats; Clams; Lobster; Shrimp; Lamb; Pheasant; various types of Crab; Chicken Wings; Abalone; Duck; Veal; Anchovy; Guinea hen; Cod; Scallops; Canned tuna; Haddock; Rabbit; Venison; Oysters; Smoked salmon; Meatless sausage; Dark Meat Turkey; Turkey Breast; Chicken breast; White Fish -- smoked; Crayfish; Croaker; Mussels; Sablefish; Flatfish (flounder & sole); Caviar; orange roughy; Pike; Perch; Calamari; Herring; Yellowfin tuna; Halibut;

Instead <u>choose</u>: Swordfish; Snapper; Ling; Sturgeon; White fish; Octopus; Catfish; Seabass; Spot; Monkfish; Tilefish; Pollock; Freshwater bass;

Eggs, Beans, Nuts and Seeds

Coconut milk; Coconut; Black-eyed peas; Lima beans; Dried coconut meat; Egg yolk; Lupin; Egg substitute; Alfalfa sprouts; Macadamia nuts; Peanuts; Egg; Lentils; Green peas;

Instead choose: various beans; Soybean seeds;

Fruits & Juices

There are no fruits that can worsen your conditions.

Vegetables

There are no vegetables that can worsen your conditions.

Breads, Grains, Cereals, Pasta

Croissant; Danish Pastry; Sweet Rolls; Donuts; Rolls including Whole-wheat, Kaiser and French; Egg Dinner Rolls; Milk crackers; Biscuits; Saltine Crackers; Chinese Noodles or Chow Mein;

Instead <u>choose</u>: Oat bran; Semolina; White bread; Spinach spaghetti; Corn muffins; Wheat; Hamburger & hot dog rolls;

Dairy Products, Fats & Oils

Margarine; Hydrogenated Vegetable Oil; Poultry fat; Margarine-like spreads; various Shortening; Salted butter; Animal Fat; various types of Vegetable/Seeds/Nut Oil; Lard; Unsalted butter; various cheese; various fish Oil; Whipped cream; Non-dairy creamers;

Instead choose: Ricotta cheese; Cheddar cheese; Colby cheese; Flaxseed oil; Sour Cream; Cod liver fish oil; Gouda cheese; Mozzarella cheese; Wheat germ oil; Cheeses: Romano, edam; Cream; Chocolate milk; Sardine fish oil;

Desserts, Snacks, Beverages

Sweet Chocolate; Chocolate Mousse; Puff Pastry; Cakes; Cookies; Éclairs; Coffee Liqueur; Pie crust; Cheesecake; Dessert Toppings; Cream Puffs; various types of Pies; Chocolate Ice Cream; after Dinner Mints; Soft (carbonated) drinks; Beer; Frostings; various candies; Pudding; 80+ Proof Alcoholic Beverages; Whiskey; Ice cream cones; Frostings; Dark chocolate; Honey; Crème de Menthe; Pancakes; various Ice Cream; Chewing Gum; Jams & Preserves; Sherbet; Fruit leather/rolls; Piña Colada; Jellies; Peanut butter; Potato sticks; Halvah;

Instead choose: Fruit punch; Lemonade; Coffee (lowers Gout risk for men); Tortilla chips; Molasses; Eggnog; Pretzels; Green tea; Applesauce; Plain tea;

Herbs & Spices, Fast Foods, Prepared Foods

Foie Gras or Liver Pate; Hot Dog; Chocolate Syrup; Chicken Nugget; Soy Sauce; Salad Dressings (e.g., French; Italian; blue/Roquefort); Beef & chicken broth; Barbecue sauce; Beef & chicken stock; various Canned Gravy; Table Salt; various sauces; Table Sugar (white or powdered); Maple syrup; Nachos; Miso; Mayonnaise; Chicken Noodle Soup; Veg/beef soup; Teriyaki Sauce; Ketchup; Capers; various Syrups; Breaded Shrimp; Fish stock; cocoa; Tabasco Sauce; various Pizza; Pickle relish; Onion Rings; Cheeseburger; Clam chowder; Sweet pickle; Sauerkraut; Mustard; Pickle;

Instead choose: Chervil; Red or cayenne pepper; Macaroni; Tomato paste; Cinnamon; Cole slaw; Black & white pepper; Turmeric; Pepper or hot sauce; Mustard seed; Mints; Saffron; Maple sugar; Poppy seed; Falafel;

Alternative Therapies & Miscellaneous

Excess body weight; 2+ alcoholic beverages/day; Corn sweetener; Fasting (i.e., do not skip meals); Smoking. Tobacco; Preparing food fried or battered; Aspirin; Preparing food smoked; High dosages of Niacin; Hyperthermia (avoid if extremely high blood pressure); Prescription drugs (diuretics such as thiazide); Stress; Salted foods, nuts, etc.

Key Nutrients & Herbal Meds

Brewer's Yeast; Caffeine; Alcohol; Saturated Fat (limit to 7% of daily calories); Licorice; Purine; Sodium/salt; Refined Sugar; Guarana; Kola (cola); Mate;

Diabetes Type 2 (& HBP)

Diabetes is a disorder that refers to our body's inability to use or convert food to the fuel needed by our cells.

Insulin is a hormone that helps the glucose (sugar) get into the body cells. In diabetes, the body is unable to create or properly use insulin. Without insulin, glucose stays in the blood and eventually makes its way to the urine, instead of serving as fuel to our muscles, tissues and brain.

There are different types of diabetes but the most common one is Diabetes Type 2 which represents 90-95% of diabetes cases, and is the focus of this section.

You are at most risk to develop diabetes Type 2 if you are obese. Your risk increases as you get older, if you are a member of a US minority group, are physically inactive, have a family history of the disease, have high blood pressure, have low level of good cholesterol, or have a high level of triglycerides.

Over time, excessive blood sugar level can cause serious health problems, in particular heart related issues. Over 65% of those with diabetes die from heart disease or stroke.

While there is no cure for diabetes type 2, there are numerous tools such as nutrition and exercise to help with the management of this disorder. In addition to managing the blood sugar level, the goal of diabetes management includes control of blood pressure, and cholesterol levels.

Choose these for Diabetes (Type 2) & High Blood Pressure

Top 5 items to consume:

Soybeans; Whole Grains; Almonds; Mushrooms; Seeds;

Food items and actions that could improve your health (within a food group, most helpful items are listed first):

Meat, Fish & Poultry

Pink salmon; Marlin; Swordfish; White fish; Trout; Carp; Snapper; Sardines; Blue fin tuna; Mackerel; Ling; Sturgeon; Catfish; Seabass; Spot; Herring; Monkfish; Tilefish; Halibut; Pollock; Bluefish; Pout; Smelt; Whiting; Freshwater bass; Perch; Yellowfin tuna; Snail; Pompano fish; Striped bass; Yellowtail; Drum; Sucker; Wolffish; Cisco (smoked); Scup; Shad; Fish roe; Milkfish; Cusk; Shark; Pike; Mullet; Eel; Tilapia; Lingcod; Sheepshead; Surimi; Grouper; Caviar; Pumpkinseed sunfish; Cisco; Rockfish; Burbot; Dolphinfish (Mahi-Mahi); Flatfish (flounder & sole); Whelk; Liver; Oysters; Cuttlefish; Chicken breast (no skin); Canned tuna; Butterfish; Seatrout; Pork loin/sirloin; Spiny lobster; Sablefish; Anchovy; Turbot; White fish (smoked); Cod; Beef filet mignon; Mussels; Beef round steak; Croaker; Veal shank; Octopus; Haddock; Ground beef; Beef rib eye; Orange roughy; Pheasant; Alaskan King crab; Beef (lean cuts); Quail (skinless); Dungeness crab; Veal (lean cuts); Pork (lean cuts); Boar meat; Chicken dark meat (skinless); Pheasant breast; Turkey breast (skinless); Bison/buffalo meat; Venison; Lamb (lean cuts); Chicken giblets; Duck (no skin); Goose; Rabbit meat; Guinea hen; Turkey dark meat (skinless); Salmon (smoked, Lox); Blue crab; Clams; Scallops; Squab (pigeon);

Eggs, Beans, Nuts and Seeds

Soybean seeds; Almonds; Hazelnuts or Filberts; Split peas; Seeds: Breadnut tree, chia, cottonseed, flaxseed, safflower, sunflower; Soy milk; Soybeans (green); Pine nuts; Pistachio nuts; Brazil nuts; Beans: navy, adzuki; Watermelon seeds; Butternuts; Black walnuts; various beans; Chickpeas; Ginkgo nuts; Pili nuts; Pumpkin & squash seeds; Cashew nuts; Walnuts; Breadfruit seeds; Peanuts; Black-eyed peas; Green peas; Sugar or snap peas; Hickory nuts; Beechnuts; Sesame seeds; Acorns; Pecans; Lupin; Alfalfa sprouts; Cornnuts; Lentils; Chestnuts; Macadamia nuts; Egg yolk; Egg white; Coconut meat (dried);

Almonds, Hazelnuts ...

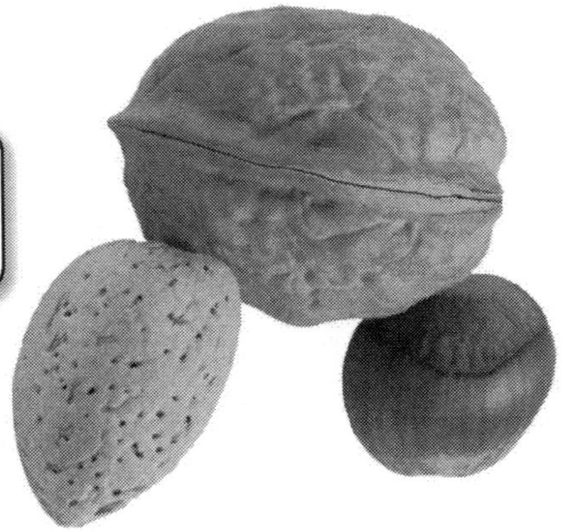

Fruits & Juices (*avoid fruit juices with added sugar or from concentrate*)

Dried prunes, peaches & apricots; Goji berry; Passion fruit; Dried banana; Elderberries; Guava; Plantains; Avocado; Apricots; Cantaloupe; Persimmons; Dried figs; Banana; Abiyuch; Raisins; Durian; Kumquats; Currants (dried); Grapefruit; Mango; Pitanga; Tamarind; Papaya; Blackberries; Raspberries; Rowal; Dried litchi; Acerola; Dates; Gooseberries; Watermelon; Jujube (fruit); Lemon; Currants (raw); Kiwi fruit; Boysenberries; Lime; dried fruits; Pears; Berries; Natal Plum (Carissa); Apples; Peaches; Breadfruit; Pumelo (Shaddock); Strawberries; Nectarine; Plum; Tangerines; Orange juice; Prune juice; Grape juice; Olives; Grapefruit juice; Pomegranate; Oranges; Apple juice; Cranberry juice; Pineapple; Blueberries and Bilberries; Figs; Honeydew melon; Cherries; Pineapple juice; Quince; Litchi; Longans; Cranberries; Pomegranate juice; Grapes; Rhubarb;

Vegetables (avoid canned vegetables)

Amaranth leaves; Fungi cloud ears; Grape leaves; Shitake mushrooms; Ancho & Pasilla peppers; Pigeon peas; Sun-dried tomatoes; Wasabi root; Taro leaves; Balsam pear leafy tips; Corn bran; Sweet potatoes leaves; Tahitian taro; Vine spinach (Basella); Chrysanthemum (Garland); Chrysanthemum Leaves; Dandelion Greens; Mustard spinach; Garden cress; Kale; Arugula; Chinese broccoli; Chicory greens; Collards; Mustard greens; Okra; Turnip greens; Bok choy; Borage; Purslane; Watercress; Winged beans leaves; Parsnips; Cauliflower; Beet greens; Broccoli; Brussels sprouts; Carrots; Endive; Green onions (scallions); Potatoes w/skin; Arrowhead; Kohlrabi; Cowpeas leafy tips; Celtuce; Hot chili peppers; Spinach; Winter squash; Quinoa seed; Yam; Nopal; Taro; Green & savoy cabbage; Green beans; Jalapeno peppers; Lambsquarters; Potato; Kelp; Portabella mushrooms; Asparagus; Bell peppers; Red cabbage; Leeks; Romaine & loose leaf lettuce; various peppers; Pokeberry shoots; Pumpkin; Pumpkin flowers; Tomatoes; Lotus root; Swiss chard; Garlic; Jew's ear mushrooms; Rutabaga; Shallots; Artichoke; Fiddlehead ferns; Sweet potatoes; Radishes; Arrowroot; Corn; Head lettuce; Yellow squash; Zucchini; Turnips; Eggplant; Sesbania Flower; Tomato juice; Hearts of palm; Celery; Onions (2-5 oz. of fresh onion daily, or 1 tsp. onion juice 3-4 times a day); other vegetables;

Breads, Grains, Cereals, Pasta

Wheat germ; Whole-wheat; Amaranth; Buckwheat; Wheat germ cereal; Durum wheat; Oats; Rye; Whole-wheat English muffins & Cereal; Triticale; Rice bran; Whole-wheat spaghetti; Sorghum; Wheat germ bread; Wheat bran muffins; Oatmeal (cereal); Spelt (cooked); Shredded wheat cereal; Whole-wheat dinner rolls; Wild rice; Granola cereal; Bulgur; Whole-grain bread; Millet; Whole-wheat crackers; Rice cakes (Brown rice based); Oat bran muffins; Pumpernickel bread; Banana bread; Tortillas (corn); Brown rice; Barley; Oat bran bread; Corn flakes; Cream of wheat; Wheat; Italian bread; Chinese chow Mein noodles; Wheat bran; Semolina; English muffins; Rice crisps cereal; White rice; Bread sticks; Corn muffins; Oat bran; Spaghetti; Pasta; Biscuits; Waffles; Bagels; Spinach spaghetti;

Dairy Products, Fats & Oils

Wheat germ oil; Cod liver fish oil; Flaxseed oil; Cheese: cottage, Gjetost, Swiss, Gruyere; Whey (dried); Salmon fish oil; Canola oil; Cheddar cheese; Walnut oil; various cheese; various fish oil; Mustard oil; Oil of: apricot kernel, hazelnut, safflower, soybean; various milk; Olive oil; other oils: almonds, grape seeds, sunflower, corn & oat; Cheese spread; Chocolate milk; Salt-free or low-salt foods

Desserts, Snacks, Beverages

Air Popped Popcorn; Sesame crunch candies; Peanut butter; Potato chips/fried snacks; Tortilla chips; Taro chips; Oil popped Popcorn; Water; Potato sticks;

Herbs & Spices, Fast Foods, Prepared Foods

Whole-grain Cornmeal; Cottonseed meal; Thyme (fresh); Tofu; Peppermint; Rosemary (fresh); Natto; Parsley; Spearmint (fresh); Dill weed; Tempeh; Basil (fresh); French fries; Coriander/Cilantro; Tomato paste; Poppy seed; Cocoa; Cayenne (red) pepper; Mustard seed; Cheese fondue; Minestrone soup; Egg rolls (veg); Corn salad; Falafel; Taco shells; Vegetable soup; Mace; Veg/beef soup; Oregano; Tarragon (dried); Succotash; Miso; Sage; Chervil; Hash brown potatoes; Cloves; Cinnamon; Pepper (black or white); Croutons; Potato pancakes; Fennel seeds; Hummus; Mints; Turmeric; Cardamom; Maple sugar;

Alternative Therapies & Miscellaneous

Consult your doctor (maintain annual physical exam, get vaccinated, monitor eyes, foot, blood pressure ...); Exercise; Follow DASH diet; Exposure to sun; Organically grown foods; Fresh (uncooked) fruits/veg's (or use no salt added canned); Biofeedback; Eat smaller, more frequent meals; Glucomannan; Meditation; Ornish Plan & Diet; Pray, practice your religion; Sleep 6-8 hours regularly; Tai Chi; Vegetarian diet; Yoga (avoid certain postures); Salt-free or low-salt foods; Consult your dentist (schedule exams twice a year);

Key Nutrients & Herbal Medicines

Siberian Ginseng; Fiber; Hawthorn (in berries form or tea from dried leaves and flowers. Do not take with other heart medications); Magnesium; Brewer's Yeast; Calcium; Celery seed; Chromium; Monounsaturated fat; Polyunsaturated fat; Gymnema; Omega-3 fatty acids; Potassium; Vitamin A; Vitamin D; Yucca; Zinc; Beta Carotene; Fenugreek seeds;

Do not choose these for High Blood Pressure & Diabetes (Type 2)

Top 5 items to avoid:

Chocolate & Sweets; 2+ alcoholic drinks/day; Hydrogenated Vegetable Oil & Animal Fat; Luncheon (processed) Meats; & Excess body weight;

Avoid or consume much less of the following (within a food group, most harmful items are listed first):

Meat, Fish & Poultry

Pepperoni; Turkey pastrami; Blood sausage; Chicken skin; Turkey skins; Beerwurst beer salami; Frankfurters; Luncheon meats; Bologna; Sausage; Salami; Pastrami; Cured beef; Chorizo; Cured meats; Pork skins; Pork liver cheese; Beef tongue; Corned beef; Beef jerky sticks; Lamb tongue;

***Instead choose:* Abalone; Crayfish; Lamb ribs; Meatless sausage; Calamari; Lobster; Bacon;**

Eggs, Beans, Nuts and Seeds

Coconut milk; Egg substitute;

Breads, Grains, Cereals, Pasta

Croissant; Danish pastry; Sweet cinnamon rolls; White bread; Donuts; Kaiser dinner rolls; Milk crackers; Saltines crackers; Sweet rolls; French rolls; Blueberry muffins;

***Instead choose:* Wheat crackers; Granola bars; Cornbread; Bran flakes cereal; Melba toasts crackers; Egg noodles; Japanese noodles; Couscous; Rice noodles; Hamburger & hot dog rolls; Matzo crackers;**

Dairy Products, Fats & Oils

Hydrogenated Vegetable oil; Animal Fat; Lard; Ucuhuba butter oil; Poultry fat; Whipped cream; Oils: Cupu Assu, Coconut, Cocoa Butter, Babassu, Shea nut; various Shortening; Non-dairy creamers; Cream; Butter (salted); Sour cream;

***Instead choose:* Peanut oil; Goat cheese; Yogurt; Skim milk; Oils: tomato seeds, cottonseed, poppy seed, rice bran; Cheese: camembert, blue, limburger, pimento, Romano;**

Desserts, Snacks, Beverages

Pound cake; Sweet chocolate; Cookies; Chocolate cake; Éclairs; Cheesecake; Cakes; Cream puffs; Dessert toppings; Vanilla cream pie; Coffee liqueur; Chocolate mousse; Puff pastry; various pies; Chocolate; Fruit leather/rolls; After-dinner mints; Ice cream; Pudding; Fruit punch; Lemonade; Soft (carbonated) drinks; Honey; Ice cream cones; Chewing gum; Jams & Preserves; Sherbet; Candies; Frozen yogurt; Jellies; Frostings; Coffeecake; Pie crust; Crème de menthe; Pancakes; Coffee; Piña colada; Dark chocolate; Plain tea; Eggnog; 80+ proof distilled alc. beverages; Whiskey; Pretzels;

***Instead choose:* Red & White wine; Peanut bar candy; Sports drinks; Beer; Tonic water; Halvah; Pumpkin pie; Herbal tea;**

Herbs & Spices, Fast Foods, Prepared Foods

Barbecue sauce; Hoisin sauce; Table sugar (white or powder); Chocolate syrup; Oyster sauce; various syrups; Hot dog; Cheese sauce; Ketchup; Italian salad dressing; Table salt; Chicken Nuggets; various sauces; Nachos; Breaded shrimp; Capers; French salad dressing; Blue/Roquefort salad dressing; Pizza; Cheeseburger; Soy sauce; Fish sauce; Nutmeg; Brown sugar; Tapioca; Macaroni; Pickle (cucumber); Potato salad; Gravies (canned);

Instead choose: Chives; Onion rings; Fish stock; Cole slaw; Saffron; Beef stock; Corn cakes; Mayonnaise; Ginger; Clam chowder; Teriyaki sauce; Sweet pickle; Marjoram; Vinegar; Chicken stock; Mustard; Beef broth; Foie gras or liver pate; Sauerkraut;

Alternative Therapies & Miscellaneous

2+ alcoholic drinks/day; Excess body weight; Smoking, tobacco; Corn sweetener; Sugared fruit juice or from concentrate; Stress; Fasting (for a specific period); Hyperthermia (if extremely high blood pressure); Processed or Refined foods; Fried or battered foods; Baking using butter; Sweeteners; Abrupt changes in diet/exercise; Aspartame (Equal); Saccharine (NutraSweet); Birth control pills; Salted foods, nuts, etc.;

Key Nutrients & Herbal Medicines

Refined sugar; Saturated fat; Caffeine; Cholesterol; Licorice; Sodium (salt); Total sugar; Trans fatty acids; Guarana; Kola (cola); Mate;

Obesity or Excess Body Weight (& HBP)

Obesity is defined as having too much body fat. It normally occurs when you continue to eat more calories than your body burns through exercise and normal daily activities. The unused calories are then stored as fat in your body leading to obesity.

Obesity is a risk factor for many diseases and illnesses including certain types of cancer. However, even a modest reduction in body fat (5 to 10% weight loss) can reduce your risk or delay illnesses caused by obesity.

The common way to measure obesity is body mass index (BMI). BMI is calculated by multiplying your weight in pounds by 703, divided by the square of your height in inches. For example a 6 feet tall man who weighs 190 pounds, has a BMI of 25.8. In the metric system, BMI is your weight in kilograms divided by the square of your height in meters.

Your BMI is considered normal if it is between 18.5 and 24.9. You are obese if your BMI is 30 or higher. You have excess body weight if your BMI is between 24.9 and 30.

Risk factors that can lead to obesity include: lack of physical exercise, overeating (e.g., oversized portions, recovery from quitting smoking), poor diet (e.g., eating high-fat foods), genetic or family history, pregnancy (inability to lose weight after giving birth), hormone problems, certain medications and illnesses, emotional issues (boredom, anger or stress), growing older, and lack of sleep.

Choose **these for High Blood Pressure & Excess Body Weight**

Top 5 items to consume:

Beans/Legumes; Rye; Soybeans; Passion fruit; <u>and Exercise</u>

Food items and actions that could improve your health (within a food group, most helpful items are listed first):

Meat, Fish & Poultry

(5.5 oz. of meat/fowl/fish or beans per day); Pink salmon; Snapper; Ling; Blue fin tuna; Seabass; Sturgeon; Monkfish; Marlin; Swordfish; White fish; Catfish; Trout; Carp; Tilefish; Halibut; Freshwater bass; Spot; Yellowfin tuna; King mackerel; Pout; Pollock; Whiting; Sucker; Wolffish; Perch; Pike; Smelt; Bluefish; Sheepshead; Cusk; Shark; Striped bass; Surimi; Snail; Lingcod; Scup; Tilapia; Burbot; Pumpkinseed sunfish; Drum; Grouper; Cisco; Rockfish; Yellowtail; Dolphinfish (Mahi-Mahi); Mullet; Herring; Turbot; Sardines; Milkfish; Cisco (smoked); Seatrout; Flatfish (flounder & sole); Cod; Fish roe; Canned tuna; Mackerel; Shad; Orange roughy; Butterfish; Haddock; Pompano fish; Chicken breast (no skin);

Eggs, Beans, Nuts and Seeds

(5.5 oz. of meat/fowl/fish or beans per day); Split peas; Beans: navy, black & pinto; Lentils; other beans; Chickpeas; Soybeans (green); Alfalfa sprouts; Black-eyed peas; Green peas; Lupin; Sugar or snap peas; Soybean seeds; Soy milk; Seeds: breadnut tree, chia, breadfruit, flaxseed; Ginkgo nuts; Almonds; Chestnuts; Safflower seeds; Hazelnuts or Filberts; Sunflower seeds;

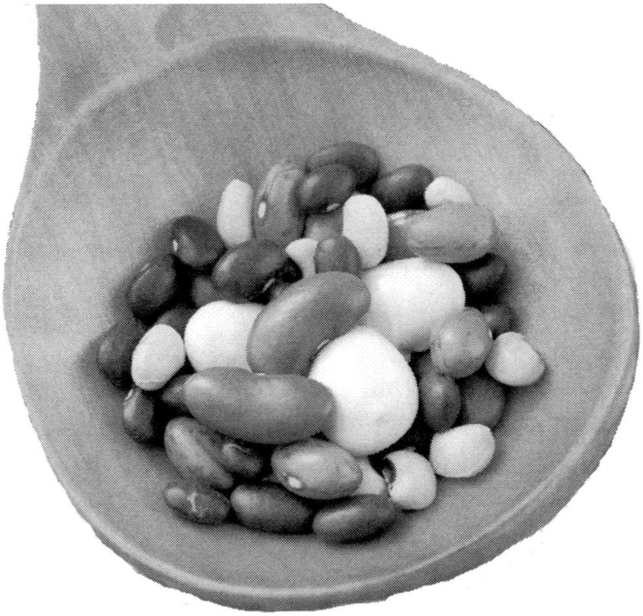

Beans / Legumes

Fruits & Juices

(2 cups of fruits & juices per day; favor fruits over juices; drink fruit juice before meals); Passion fruit; Elderberries; Dried figs; Abiyuch; Guava; Prunes (dried); Dried peaches; Blackberries; Raspberries; Durian; Banana; Berries; Kumquats; Tamarind; Dried banana & apricots; Currants (raw); Kiwi fruit; Rowal; Goji berry; Raisins; Currants (dried); Lemon; Lime; Pears; Breadfruit; Grape juice; Jujube (fruit); Natal Plum (Carissa); Persimmons; Prune juice; Dates; Dried fruits; Cranberry juice; Apricots; Cantaloupe; Pomegranate; Plantains; Apple juice; Grapefruit juice; Orange juice; Avocado; Acerola; Pitanga; Pumelo (Shaddock); Strawberries; Figs; Peaches; Blueberries and Bilberries; Grapefruit; Honeydew melon; Nectarine; Oranges; Papaya; Pineapple; Plum; Watermelon; Apples; Cherries; Mango; Pomegranate juice; Quince; Tangerines; Longans; Grapes; Litchi; Pineapple juice; Cranberries; Rhubarb; Olives;

Vegetables

(2.5 cups per day); Corn bran; Fungi cloud ears; Ancho peppers; Pigeon peas; Grape leaves; Pasilla peppers; Wasabi root; Shitake mushrooms; Sweet potatoes leaves; Epazote; Artichoke; Taro leaves; Garlic; Amaranth leaves; Arrowhead; Potatoes w/skin; Quinoa seed; Chrysanthemum (Garland); Chrysanthemum Leaves; Dandelion Greens; Mustard spinach; Yam; Balsam pear leafy tips; Sun-dried tomatoes; Tahitian taro; Vine spinach (Basella); Taro; Chinese broccoli; Chicory greens; Collards; Mustard greens; Okra; Turnip greens; Garden cress; Kale; Arugula; Kelp; Nopal; Lotus root; Parsnips; Beet greens; Balsam pear; Broccoli; Brussels sprouts; Carrots; Endive; Green onions (scallions); Kohlrabi; Jalapeno peppers; Bok choy; Borage; Cowpeas leafy tips; Purslane; Watercress; Winged beans leaves; Shallots; Onions (2-5 oz. of fresh onion daily, or 1 tsp. onion juice 3-4 times a day); Potato; Cauliflower; Green & Savoy cabbage; Eggplant; Green beans; various peppers; Fiddlehead ferns; Arrowroot; Portabella mushrooms; Celtuce; Rutabaga; Spinach; various squash; Zucchini; Corn; Jerusalem Artichoke; Beets; Asparagus; Bell peppers; other vegetables;

Breads, Grains, Cereals, Pasta

(6 oz. of grains per day with over 3 oz. from whole grains); Rye; Durum wheat; Buckwheat; Amaranth; Oats; Whole-wheat cereal; Wheat germ cereal; Sorghum; Spelt (cooked); Whole-wheat spaghetti; Whole-wheat bread; Triticale; Barley; Bulgur; Whole-wheat English muffins; Oatmeal (cereal); Millet; Brown rice; Rice bran; Wild rice; Shredded wheat cereal; Wheat bran; Whole-wheat; Bran flakes cereal; Wheat germ bread; Tortillas (corn); Whole-wheat dinner rolls; White rice; Wheat germ; Oat bran muffins; Oat bran; Wheat bran muffins;

Dairy Products, Fats & Oils

(3 cups of low fat products per day); Fat-free/Low fat, low salt dairy products; Cottage cheese; Milk;

Desserts, Snacks, Beverages

Air-popped Popcorn; Water (6 to 8 8 oz. glasses per day); Red wine; White wine;

Herbs & Spices, Fast Foods, Prepared Foods

Thyme (fresh); Whole-grain Cornmeal; Peppermint; Rosemary (fresh); Tofu; Natto; Cottonseed meal; Spearmint (fresh); Parsley; Tempeh; Dill weed; Succotash; Coriander/Cilantro; Fennel seeds; Oregano; Sage; Basil (fresh); Tarragon (dried); Cayenne (red) pepper; Cinnamon; Pepper (black or white); Turmeric;

Alternative Therapies & Miscellaneous

Exercise (include sit-ups and lower back exercises); Fat-free or low fat products; Walk, wheel, or jog (such stomach in while running); Follow DASH diet; Salt-free or low-salt foods; Choose smaller food portions, take smaller meals; Fresh (uncooked) fruits/veg's or use no salt added canned; Hang mirrors where you eat; Hypnotherapy; Meditation; Ornish Plan & Diet; Pray, practice your religion; Sleep 6-8 hours regularly; Tai Chi; Vegetarian diet; Yoga (certain postures must be avoided); Organically grown foods;

Key Nutrients & Herbal Medicines

Fiber; Hawthorn (in berries form or tea from dried leaves and flowers. Do not take with other heart medications); Calcium; Celery seed; Siberian Ginseng; Magnesium; Potassium; Yucca;

<u>Do not</u> choose these for High Blood Pressure & Excess Body Weight

Top 5 items to avoid:

2+ alcoholic drinks/day; Chocolate & Sweets; Luncheon (processed) Meats; Margarine & Hydrogenated vegetable oil; Salad dressings;

Avoid or consume much less of the following (within a food group, most harmful items are listed first):

Meat, Fish & Poultry

Chorizo; Frankfurters; Luncheon (processed) meats; Pepperoni; Pork liver cheese; Pork skins; Salamis; Sausages; Bacon; Cured beef; Pastrami; Beef jerky sticks; Cured meats; Bologna; Chicken skin; Turkey skins; Beef chuck/brisket; Beef/Lamb tongue; Beef ribs; Pork ribs; Lamb ribs; Pork; Lamb; Beef; Pork headcheese; Lamb; Squab (pigeon); Corned beef; Pancreas (lamb, beef, veal); Bison/buffalo meat; Goose; Organ meats; Liver; Chicken dark meat; Chicken wings; Shrimp; Clams; Caviar; Abalone; Veal loin; Veal; Lobster; Beef/Lamb brain; Beef filet mignon; Quail; Alaskan King crab; Rabbit meat; Salmon (smoked, Lox); Calamari; Venison; Eel;

Instead <u>choose</u>: Whelk; White fish (smoked); Mussels; Turkey breast; Spiny lobster; Oysters; Octopus; Quail breast; Cuttlefish; Pheasant breast; Crayfish; Dungeness crab; Turkey dark meat; Guinea hen; Scallops;

Eggs, Beans, Nuts and Seeds

Coconut milk; Egg yolk; Coconut; Macadamia nuts; Coconut meat (dried); Egg substitute; Egg; Hickory nuts; Pecans; Egg white; Beechnuts;

Instead <u>choose</u>: Black walnuts; Pistachio nuts; Butternuts; Cottonseed; Sesame seeds; Pine nuts;

Breads, Grains, Cereals, Pasta

Croissant; Saltines crackers; Sweet rolls; Milk crackers; Donuts; Wheat crackers; Rice crisps cereal; Danish pastry; Granola bars; Biscuits; Blueberry muffins; Kaiser rolls; French rolls; Bread sticks; Melba toasts crackers; Chinese chow Mein noodles; Corn flakes; Matzo crackers; White bread; Waffles; Granola cereal; Hamburger & hot dog rolls; Banana bread; Cornbread;

Instead <u>choose</u>: Pumpernickel bread; English muffins; Pasta; Spaghetti; Rice cakes (Brown rice based); Spinach spaghetti;

Dairy Products, Fats & Oils

Margarine (salted); Margarine-like spreads; Hydrogenated vegetable Oil; Margarine (unsalted); Butter (salted); Animal fat; Oils: Babassu, Cocoa Butter, cottonseed, Cupu Assu, palm, peanut, poppy seed, rice bran, sesame, Shea nut, tea seed, Ucuhuba Butter; Brie cheese; Lard; other seeds/nuts/vegetable oils; Vegetable shortening; poultry fats; Cheeses: Roquefort, goat, pimento, feta, camembert; Butter (unsalted); Other cheese; Whipped cream; Cheese spread; Sour cream; Non-dairy creamers; Various fish oil; Wheat germ oil; Salmon fish oil;

Instead choose: Whey (dried); Yogurt; low fat and low salt versions of cheese;

Desserts, Snacks, Beverages

Pound cake; Sweet chocolate; Cookies; Puff pastry; Pie crust; Chocolate cake; Éclairs; Cheesecake; various cakes; Cream puffs; Dessert toppings; Coffeecake; Vanilla cream pie; Chocolate mousse; various pies; Fruit leather/rolls; After-dinner mints; Ice creams; Peanut brittle candy; Frostings; Ice cream cones; Potato sticks; Fruit punch; Lemonade; Pretzels; Honey; Chewing gum; Jams & Preserves; Pancakes; Coffee liqueur; Sherbet; various candies; Pudding; Frozen yogurt; Taro chips; Jellies; Soft (carbonated) drinks; Tortilla chips; Oil popped popcorn; Halvah; Peanut butter; Dark chocolate; Crème de menthe; Potato chips/fried snacks; Coffee; Hot chocolate; Piña colada;

Instead choose: Tonic water; Beer; Sports drinks; Sesame crunch candies; Herbal tea; Ginger ale; Green tea;

Herbs & Spices, Fast Foods, Prepared Foods

Salad dressings: blue/Roquefort, French, Italian; Foie gras or liver pate; Sauces: Hoisin, Sofrito, oyster; Hot dog; Barbecue sauce; Mayonnaise; various sauce; Table sugar (white or powder); Chicken Nuggets; Soy sauce; Chocolate syrup; Nachos; Pizza; Ketchup; Table salt; various syrups; Breaded shrimp; Onion rings; Tabasco sauce; Capers; Cheeseburger; Tapioca; Hash brown potatoes; Teriyaki sauce; French toast; Potato pancakes; Brown sugar; Corn cakes; Potato salad; Macaroni; Hamburger; Maple sugar; Taco shells; Pickle relish; Croutons; Hush puppies; Pickle (cucumber); Falafel; Mustard; Gravies (canned); Beef broth; Chicken broth; Chicken noodle soup; Veg/beef soup; Sweet pickle; Miso; Nutmeg;

Instead choose: Poppy seed; Chervil; Cocoa; French fries; Mace; Mustard seed; Corn salad; Mints; Saffron; Fish stock; Cloves; Tomato paste; Molasses; Chives; Couscous; Ginger; Marjoram; Vinegar; Cardamom; Egg rolls (veg); Clam chowder;

Alternative Therapies & Miscellaneous

2+ alcoholic drinks/day; Corn sweetener; Sugared fruit juice or from concentrate; Stress; Processed or Refined foods; Fried or battered foods[7]; Salted foods, nuts, etc.; Hyperthermia (avoid if extremely high blood pressure); Smoking, tobacco; Baking using butter; Sweeteners;

Key Nutrients & Herbal Medicines

Refined Sugar; Saturated Fat (limit to 7% of daily calories); Sodium/salt (limit to 1500 mg per day); Caffeine; Total fat; Licorice;

Daily calorie intake should be limited to 10 for each pound of your desired weight, e.g., for a desired weight of 160 lbs., consume 1,600 calories per day.

Depression (& HBP)

Depression is a serious chronic illness. It is not just a temporary feeling of being down. It is a disorder of the brain. It can interfere with your normal life and lead to various physical and emotional problems. It affects men, women and elderly in different ways.

The exact cause of depression is unknown. But several factors can lead to depression: loss of a loved one, stressful situations such as a difficult relationship or financial problems, family history of depression (genetic factors), differences in brain chemistry, changes in body hormones, and traumatic events during one's childhood.

You are more likely to get depression if you are between 15 and 30 years old, you are a woman, it is winter time, or it is just after you gave birth to a baby.

Choose these for High Blood Pressure & Depression

Top 5 items to consume:

Soybeans; Whole Grains; Seeds; Fish; Walnuts;

Food items and actions that could improve your health (within a food group, most helpful items are listed first):

Meat, Fish & Poultry

Pink salmon; Fish roe; Marlin; Swordfish; Trout; White fish; Blue fin tuna; Mackerel; Ling; Spot; Sardines; Herring; Tilefish; Bluefish; Seabass; Whelk; Striped bass; Pollock; Carp; Snapper; Caviar; Milkfish; Smelt; Monkfish; Pompano fish; Wolffish; Walleye pike; Mussels; Shad; Yellowtail; Drum; Shark; Freshwater bass; Yellowfin tuna; Pout; Scup; Whiting; Cisco (smoked); Sucker; Sturgeon; Snail; Liver; Octopus; Halibut; Cuttlefish; Anchovy; Perch; Burbot; Catfish; Calamari; Mullet; Lingcod; Chicken giblets; Sheepshead; Beef brain; Spiny lobster; Pork liver; Surimi; Cusk; Pork/Veal kidneys; Rockfish; Grouper; Dolphinfish (Mahi-Mahi); Sablefish; Pork loin/sirloin; Cisco; Butterfish; Pumpkinseed sunfish; Tilapia; Dungeness crab; Northern pike; Eel; Chicken breast (no skin); Seatrout; Venison; Turbot; Flatfish (flounder & sole); Beef/Lamb/Veal heart; Crayfish; Clams; Beef spleen; Canned tuna; Alaskan King crab; Turkey breast; Pork leg/ham; Rabbit meat; Blue crab; Pheasant; Haddock; Cod; Quail breast; Beef filet mignon; Veal shank; White fish (smoked); Boar meat; Scallops; Orange roughy; Duck (no skin); Oysters; Turkey dark meat; Veal loin; Quail; Beef round steak; Shrimp; Veal; Abalone; Beef; Croaker; Guinea hen; Lamb leg; Meatless sausage;

Eggs, Beans, Nuts and Seeds

Soybean seeds; Split peas; Seeds: chia, cottonseed, flaxseed, safflower, sunflower; Soy milk; Walnuts; Soybeans (green); Pistachio nuts; Almonds; Peanuts; Hazelnuts or Filberts; Butternuts; Ginkgo nuts; Beans: pinto, navy; Breadfruit seeds; Breadnut tree seeds; Lentils; Pine nuts; Sesame seeds; various beans; Chickpeas; Watermelon seeds; Beechnuts; Brazil nuts; Cashew nuts; Pili nuts; Black-eyed peas; Pumpkin & squash seeds; Green peas; Chestnuts; Lupin; Hickory nuts; Egg yolk; Sugar or snap peas; Alfalfa sprouts; Acorns; Pecans; Egg; Egg white; Cornnuts; Macadamia nuts;

Fruits & Juices

Goji berry; dried Banana & Litchi; Tamarind; Prunes (dried); Currants (dried); dried Longans; Raisins; Dried fruits: Figs, Peaches, Apricots; Durian; Dates; Banana; Prune juice; Pineapple juice; Plantains; Passion fruit; other dried fruits; Elderberries; Guava; Avocado; Grape juice; Abiyuch; Cranberry juice; Boysenberries; Breadfruit; Currants (raw); Kiwi fruit; Pears; Apricots; Blackberries; Cantaloupe; Jujube (fruit); Kumquats; various berries; Longans; Natal Plum (Carissa); Persimmons; Rowal; Apple juice; Grapefruit juice; Orange juice; Mango; Figs; Lemon; Lime; Pomegranate; Apples; Grapes; Peaches; Acerola; Blueberries and Bilberries; Cherries; Grapefruit; Honeydew melon; Litchi; Nectarine; Oranges; Papaya; Pineapple; Pitanga; Plum; Pomegranate juice; Pumelo (Shaddock); Quince; Strawberries; Tangerines; Watermelon; (***use fresh/uncooked fruits***)

Vegetables

Shitake mushrooms; Pasilla peppers; Pigeon peas; Ancho peppers; Sun-dried tomatoes; Balsam pear leafy tips; Epazote; Fungi cloud ears; Garlic; Taro leaves; Winged beans leaves; Grape leaves; Chrysanthemum (Garland); Chrysanthemum Leaves; Sweet potatoes leaves; Amaranth leaves; Vine spinach (Basella); Garden cress; Wasabi root; Arrowhead; Potatoes w/skin; Dandelion Greens; Mustard spinach; Corn bran; Arrowroot; Kelp; Cowpeas leafy tips; Tahitian taro; Turnip greens; Artichoke; Collards; Kale; Spinach; Quinoa seed; Arugula; Okra; Yam; Chinese broccoli; Chicory greens; Mustard greens; Red hot chili peppers; Taro; Lambsquarters; Nopal; Brussels sprouts; Endive; Bok choy; Potato; Lotus root; Cauliflower; Broccoli; Shallots; various peppers; Parsnips; Beet greens; Borage; Purslane; Beets; Asparagus; Balsam pear; Green onions (scallions); Kohlrabi; Savoy cabbage; Watercress; Jerusalem artichoke; Portabella mushrooms; Onions (2-5 oz. of fresh onion daily, or 1 tsp. onion juice 3-4 times a day); Celtuce; Squash; Zucchini; Carrots; Romaine lettuce; Fiddlehead ferns; Corn; Rutabaga; Red bell peppers; Leeks; Pokeberry shoots; Sesbania Flower; Green cabbage; various mushrooms; other vegetables; (***use fresh/uncooked vegetables***)

Soybeans

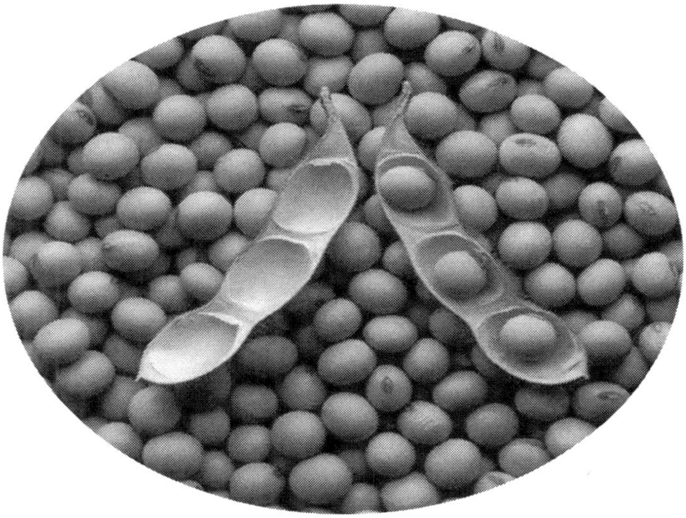

Breads, Grains, Cereals, Pasta

Wheat bran; Wheat germ; Wheat germ cereal; Amaranth; Whole-wheat; Wheat germ bread; Bran flakes cereal; Durum wheat; Rice bran; Buckwheat; Oats; Whole-wheat cereal; Whole-wheat bread; Rye; Triticale; Shredded wheat cereal; Whole-wheat English muffins; Wheat bran muffins; Whole-wheat spaghetti; Oatmeal (cereal); Granola cereal; Sorghum; Whole-wheat dinner rolls; Oat bran bread; Oat bran muffins; Spelt (cooked); Brown rice; Whole-wheat crackers; Millet; Pumpernickel bread; Barley; Bulgur; Italian bread; Wild rice; Corn flakes; Hamburger & hot dog rolls; Cornbread; Rice cakes (Brown rice based); Bread sticks; Rice crisps; Corn muffins; Banana bread; Wheat crackers; Semolina; Tortillas (corn); White rice; White bread; Waffles; Pasta; English muffins; Cream of wheat; Melba toasts crackers; Chinese chow Mein noodles; Matzo crackers; Spaghetti;

Dairy Products, Fats & Oils

Whey (dried); Wheat germ oil; Cod liver fish oil; Gjetost cheese; various fish oil; Flaxseed oil; Cheeses: cottage, Swiss, gruyere; Milk; Cheeses: cheddar, Colby; Yogurt;

Desserts, Snacks, Beverages

Air-popped Popcorn; Sesame crunch candies; Molasses; Peanut butter; Halvah candies; Potato chips/fried snacks; Water; Milk shakes;

Herbs & Spices, Fast Foods, Prepared Foods

Cottonseed meal; Tofu; Whole-grain cornmeal; Tempeh; Thyme (fresh); Peppermint; Natto; Rosemary (fresh); Cheese fondue; Miso; Cocoa; Teriyaki sauce; Dill weed; French fries; Spearmint (fresh); Parsley; Sorghum syrup; Tarragon (dried); Croutons; Sage; Basil (fresh); Succotash; Hamburger; Chervil; Oregano; Falafel; Coriander/Cilantro; Egg rolls (veg); Malt syrup; Potato pancakes; Tomato paste; Taco shells; Poppy seed; Fennel seeds; Cayenne (red) pepper;

Alternative Therapies & Miscellaneous

Exercise; Follow DASH diet; Meditation; Ornish Plan & Diet; Pray, practice your religion; Sleep 6-8 hours regularly; Tai Chi; Fresh (uncooked) fruits/veg's or no salt added canned; Biofeedback; Exposure to sun (in winter use sun lamp); Fat-free or low fat products; Hypnotherapy; Socialize, join a club; Sound Therapy; Yoga (avoid certain postures); Salt-free or low-salt foods; Organically grown foods;

Key Nutrients & Herbal Medicines

Hawthorn (in berries form or tea from dried leaves and flowers. Do not take with other heart medications); Omega-3 fatty acids; Magnesium; Calcium; Celery seed; DHEA (dehydroepiandosterone); Ginkgo Biloba; Siberian Ginseng; Potassium; SAMe (works best with Vitamin B12 and Folic acid); St. John's wort (a dose of 2-4 grams of the herb for a mild antidepressant action or nervous disturbances); Valerian (don't combine with alcohol); Yucca;

Do not choose these for High Blood Pressure & Depression

Top 5 items to avoid:

2+ Alcoholic drinks/day; Margarine & Hydrogenated Oil; Smoking; Chocolate; Various Oils & animal fat;

Avoid or consume much less of the following (within a food group, most harmful items are listed first):

Meat, Fish & Poultry

Blood sausage; Beef and pork frankfurters; Luncheon (processed) meats; Beerwurst beer salami; Cured meats; Pork skins; Cured beef; Pepperoni; various sausages; Pastrami; Chicken skin; Chorizo; Bologna; Bacon; Salami; Chicken & turkey frankfurters; Turkey skins; Beef jerky sticks; Pork liver cheese; Beef ribs; Pork headcheese;

Instead choose: Pork spare ribs; Pork back ribs; Lobster; Beef tenderloin/Tbone/portrhse; Pork cured/ham; Bison/buffalo meat; Goose; Salmon (smoked, Lox); Chicken dark meat; Chicken wings; Lamb;

Eggs, Beans, Nuts and Seeds

Coconut milk;

Instead choose: Egg substitute

Breads, Grains, Cereals, Pasta

Croissant; Danish pastry; Donuts;

Instead choose: Oat bran; Bagels; Wheat; Spinach spaghetti; Saltines crackers; French rolls; Granola bars; Egg noodles; Couscous; Rice noodles; Milk crackers; Biscuits;

Dairy Products, Fats & Oils

Hydrogenated vegetable Oil; Margarine; Margarine-like spreads; Animal fat; Oils: Babassu, Cocoa Butter, cottonseed, Cupu Assu, palm, peanut, poppy seed, rice bran, sesame, Shea nut, tea seed, Ucuhuba Butter; Lard; various seeds/nuts/vegetable oils; Vegetable shortening; Poultry fats; Butter; Whipped cream; Cream cheese; Cream; Non-dairy creamers;

Instead choose: Cheeses: port de salut, Romano, mozzarella, ricotta, gouda, parmesan; Chocolate milk; other cheese; Canola oil; Walnut oil; Cheese spread; Sour cream;

Desserts, Snacks, Beverages

Chocolate chip cookies; Sweet chocolate; Chocolate cake; Butter cookies; Pound cake; Dessert toppings; Coffee liqueur; Chocolate mousse; Pie crust; Cheesecake; Cookies; various cookies; Puff pastry; various cakes; 80+ proof distilled alc. bev.; Whiskey; After-dinner mints; Coconut cream pie; Éclairs; Coffeecake; Vanilla cream pie; Crème de menthe; Cream puffs; various pies; Piña colada; Chocolate ice cream; Pudding; Fruit leather/rolls; Peanut brittle candies; Fruit punch; Lemonade; Soft (carbonated) drinks; Potato sticks; Honey; Frostings;

Instead choose: Pretzels; Dark chocolate; Frozen yogurt; Tonic water; Ice cream cones; Tortilla chips; Oil popped popcorn; Malted drinks (nonalcoholic); Sports drinks; Eggnog; Peanut bar candies; Applesauce; Ginger ale; Herbal tea;

Herbs & Spices, Fast Foods, Prepared Foods

Salad dressings: Blue/Roquefort, French; Table salt; Oyster sauce; Chocolate syrup; Italian salad dressing; Hoisin sauce; Foie gras or liver pate; Mayonnaise; various sauces; Barbecue sauce; Capers; Table sugar (white or powder); Ketchup; Tabasco sauce; Hot dog; Chicken Nuggets; Nachos; Breaded shrimp; Syrup (table blends); Onion rings; Pickle relish; Pickle (cucumber); Gravies (canned);

Instead choose: Mustard seed; Soy sauce; Pepper (black or white); Turmeric; Cheeseburger; Corn cakes; Hush puppies; Beef stock; Corn salad; Mints; Saffron; Cinnamon; Fish stock; Maple sugar; Maple syrup; Cardamom; Mace; Clam chowder; Beef broth; Veg/beef soup; Hummus; Cloves; Chives; Ginger; Marjoram; Brown sugar; Vinegar; Chicken stock; Minestrone soup; Horseradish; Sweet pickle;

Alternative Therapies & Miscellaneous

2+ alcoholic drinks/day; Smoking, tobacco; Excess body weight; Stress; Hyperthermia (avoid if extremely high blood pressure); Salted foods, nuts, etc.; Birth control pills; Corn sweetener; Fruit juice, sugared/concentrate;

Key Nutrients & Herbal Medicines

Alcohol; Licorice; Marijuana; Sodium/salt (limit to 1500 mg per day); Saturated fat;

Alzheimer's Disease (& HBP)

Dementia is a brain disorder that refers to our loss of ability to think, remember, reason and perform daily activities. Among people older than 60, Alzheimer's Disease (AD) is the most common cause of dementia.

AD causes the gradual decline and loss of brain cells and the ability for cells (neuron) to communicate with each other. Thus a person affected with AD, has fewer brain cells and fewer connections among the brain's remaining cells. This results in a steady decline in our memory (as in remembering people's names, or doing daily tasks), and cognitive functions such as reasoning.

A combination of factors is believed to cause AD. Among these risk factors are: age (starting at the age of 60 and increasing over time), immediate family history of AD, sex (women are more likely than men to develop AD), and the same risk factors associated with heart disease (i.e., high blood pressure, high cholesterol, diabetes, lack of exercise and smoking). Higher levels of on-going intellectual and social activities have been found to reduce the risk of developing AD.

There is neither a proven approach to prevent nor to cure this disease. But there is some evidence that reducing risk of high blood pressure, high cholesterol, obesity and diabetes can reduce the risk of developing AD. Therefore, proper nutrition, exercise and staying mentally and socially active can all play an important role.

Choose these for High Blood Pressure & Alzheimer's Disease

Top 5 items to consume:

Wheat germ; Fish & fish roe; Soybeans & Soy products; Whole wheat & Amaranth; Exercise;

Food items and actions that could improve your health (within a food group, most helpful items are listed first):

Meat, Fish & Poultry

Pink salmon; Fish roe; Marlin; Swordfish; White fish; Trout; Blue fin tuna; Sardines; Ling; Mackerel; Snapper; Sturgeon; Carp; Seabass; Herring; Spot; Cisco (smoked); Monkfish; Tilefish; Caviar; Bluefish; Striped bass; Catfish; Pollock; Pompano fish; Whiting; Smelt; Freshwater bass; Snail; Walleye pike; Shark; Pout; Drum; Sucker; Wolffish; Milkfish; Scup; King mackerel; Halibut; Yellowtail; Perch; Anchovy; Shad; Rockfish; Mullet; Lingcod; Surimi; Yellowfin tuna; Chicken liver; Tilapia; White fish (smoked); Sheepshead; Grouper; Flatfish (flounder & sole); Northern pike; Cisco; Burbot; Cusk; Dolphinfish (Mahi-Mahi); Mussels; Beef brain; Whelk; Pumpkinseed sunfish; Seatrout; Liver; Turbot; Sablefish; Orange roughy; Eel; Cod; Butterfish; Calamari; Crayfish; Haddock; Octopus; Canned tuna; Chicken breast (no skin); Cuttlefish; Spiny lobster; Salmon (smoked, Lox); Chicken & Turkey giblets; Crabs: blue, Dungeness; Croaker;

Eggs, Beans, Nuts and Seeds

Soy milk; Soybeans (green); Soybean seeds; Split peas; Breadnut tree seeds; Almonds; Hazelnuts or Filberts; Seeds: chia, flaxseed, sunflower; Pinto beans; Chickpeas; Lentils; Beans: Mung, navy, moth beans, kidney, adzuki, fava; Sugar or snap peas; Black-eyed peas; various beans; Ginkgo nuts; Egg white; Green peas; Peanuts; Breadfruit seeds; Egg yolk; Pine nuts; Egg; Walnuts; Alfalfa sprouts; Chestnuts; Lupin; Safflower seeds; Pistachio nuts; Cottonseed; Brazil nuts; Butternuts;

Fruits & Juices

Dried Litchi, Apricots, Prunes; Raisins; dried banana; Tamarind; dried figs, Peaches, Currants; Guava; Goji berry; Dates; dried Longans; Abiyuch; Passion fruit; Currants (raw); Kiwi fruit; Pineapple juice; Jujube (fruit); Longans; Persimmons; Elderberries; dried fruits; Prune juice; Orange juice; Grape juice; Kumquats; Lemon; Banana; Avocado; Cantaloupe; Natal Plum (Carissa); Acerola; Breadfruit; Litchi; Oranges; Papaya; Pumelo (Shaddock); Strawberries; Cranberry juice; Grapefruit juice; Boysenberries; Pears; Mango; Pineapple; Plantains; Apricots; various berries; Rowal; Durian; Apple juice; Lime; Figs; Pomegranate; Apples; Grapes; Peaches; Grapefruit; Cherries; Nectarine; Plum; Pomegranate juice; Watermelon; Pitanga; Tangerines; Honeydew melon; Quince; Rhubarb;

Vegetables

Taro leaves; Balsam pear leafy tips; Turnip greens; Vine spinach (Basella); Amaranth leaves; Mustard spinach; Sun-dried tomatoes; Dandelion Greens; Garden cress; Collards; Tahitian taro; Mustard greens; Grape leaves; Kale; Epazote; Wasabi root; Pigeon peas; Jalapeno peppers; Garlic; Spinach; Chicory greens; Chrysanthemum (Garland); Chrysanthemum Leaves; Broccoli; Balsam pear; Bok choy; Brussels sprouts; Cowpeas leafy tips; Pasilla peppers; Cauliflower; Artichoke; Arugula; Red bell peppers; Kohlrabi; Watercress; Shitake mushrooms; Hot chili peppers; Arrowhead; Kelp; Arrowroot; Sweet potatoes leaves; Beet greens; Fungi cloud ears; Okra; Sesbania Flower; Borage; Ancho peppers; Winged beans leaves; Taro; Lambsquarters; various peppers; Nopal; Potatoes w/skin; various cabbages; Green bell peppers; Endive; Fiddlehead ferns; Pokeberry shoots; Purslane; Lotus root; Parsnips; Asparagus; Yam; Green onions (scallions); Quinoa seed; Beets; Celtuce; Rutabaga; Pumpkin flowers; Onions (2-5 oz. of fresh onion daily, or 1 tsp. onion juice 3-4 times a day); Swiss chard; Yellow squash; Zucchini; Carrots; Romaine lettuce; Shallots; Jerusalem artichoke; various mushrooms; Winter squash; Leeks; Radishes; Eggplant; Green beans; Potato; Cucumbers with peel; various lettuce; Pumpkin; Tomatoes; Turnips; Tomato juice; Hearts of palm; Celery; Fennel;

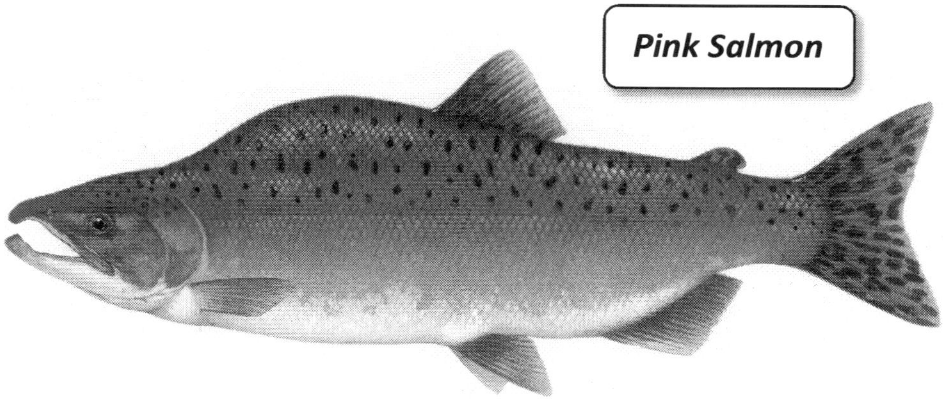

Breads, Grains, Cereals, Pasta

Wheat germ cereal; Wheat germ; Whole-wheat Bread; Amaranth Whole-wheat English Muffins;; Whole-wheat; Buckwheat; Rye; Durum wheat; Corn bran; Whole-wheat Cereal; Oats; Sorghum; Triticale; Whole-wheat Spaghetti; Oatmeal (cereal); Wheat Germ Bread; Spelt (cooked); Millet; Brown rice; Barley; Bulgur; Whole-wheat Dinner Rolls; Corn; Bran flakes cereal; Wild rice; Wheat bran; Granola cereal; Oat bran muffins; Whole-wheat crackers; Rice bran; Shredded wheat cereal; Wheat bran muffins; Oat bran bread;

Dairy Products, Fats & Oils

Wheat Germ Oil; Whey (dried); Cod Liver Fish Oil; various fish oil; Canola oil; Flaxseed oil; Cottage cheese; Fat-free or Low Fat products;

Desserts, Snacks, Beverages

Air-popped Popcorn; Molasses; Sesame crunch candies; Water;

Herbs & Spices, Fast Foods, Prepared Foods

Tofu; Whole-grain Cornmeal; Thyme (fresh); Tempeh; Peppermint; Parsley; Cottonseed meal; Dill weed; Miso; Rosemary (fresh); Tomato paste; Teriyaki sauce; Natto; Spearmint (fresh); Coriander/Cilantro; Oregano; Tarragon (dried); Sorghum syrup; Cheese fondue; Basil (fresh); Sage; Corn salad; Cayenne (red) pepper; Succotash; Fennel seeds;

Alternative Therapies & Miscellaneous

Exercise; Follow DASH diet; Fresh (uncooked) fruits/veg's or use no salt added canned; Fat-free or low fat products; Exposure to sun; Challenge your mind (with puzzles, games, books); L-carnitine (available as a dietary supplement); Meditation; Ornish Plan & Diet; Pray, practice your religion; Sleep 6-8 hours regularly; Tai Chi; Yoga (certain postures must be avoided); Salt-free or low-salt foods; Organically grown foods;

Key Nutrients & Herbal Medicines

Hawthorn (in berries form or tea from dried leaves and flowers. Do not take with other heart medications); Omega-3 fatty acids; Calcium; Celery seed; Ginkgo Biloba (Standardized Leaf extract); Siberian Ginseng; Magnesium; Potassium; Vitamin D; Vitamin E (Tocopherol); Yucca;

Do not choose these for High Blood Pressure & Alzheimer's Disease

Top 5 items to avoid:

Cured & Luncheon Meats; Hydrogenated Vegetable Oil; Sweet chocolate; 2+ Alcoholic drinks/day; Fats & Oils;

Avoid or consume much less of the following (within a food group, most harmful items are listed first):

Meat, Fish & Poultry

Cured beef; Bacon; Chorizo; various sausage; Pork skins; Luncheon meats; Pepperoni; Pork liver cheese; various salami; Frankfurters; Bologna; Beef chuck/brisket; Beef jerky sticks; Beef ribs; Pastrami; Pork ribs; Lamb ribs; Chicken skin; Turkey skins; Cured meats; Lamb/Beef tongue; Ground lamb; Pork spare ribs; Bison/buffalo meat; Lamb; Beef; Pork; Pork headcheese; Corned beef; Meatless sausage; Squab (pigeon); Organ meats; Veal; Chicken dark meat; Goose; Chicken wings;

Instead choose: Turkey breast; Shrimp; Scallops; Abalone; Pheasant breast; Turkey dark meat; Pheasant; Clams; Oysters; Guinea hen; Quail breast; Alaskan king crab; Duck (no skin);

Eggs, Beans, Nuts and Seeds

Coconut milk; Coconut meat (dried); Coconut; Macadamia nuts; Egg substitute; Pecans;

Instead choose: Beechnuts; Cornnuts; Acorns; Pili nuts; Cashew nuts;

Breads, Grains, Cereals, Pasta

Croissant; Saltines crackers; Danish pastry; Donuts; Milk crackers; Sweet rolls; Wheat crackers; Biscuits; Blueberry muffins; Granola bars; Waffles; Kaiser dinner rolls; French rolls; Chinese chow Mein noodles;

Instead choose: Semolina; Tortillas (corn); Rice cakes (Brown rice based); Breads: pumpernickel, Italian; Oat bran; Corn flakes; White rice; Spinach spaghetti; Corn muffins; Wheat;

Dairy Products, Fats & Oils

Hydrogenated vegetable oil; Animal fat; Oils: Cupu Assu, sesame, Shea nut, tea seed, Ucuhuba Butter; Brie cheese; Cocoa Butter oil; Lard; Avocado oil; Margarine; Pimento cheese; Margarine-like spreads; Parmesan cheese; various cheeses; Butter (salted); Whipped cream; various seeds/nuts/vegetable oils; Cream; Vegetable shortening; Poultry fats; Butter (unsalted); Sour cream; Chocolate milk; Non-dairy creamers; Gjetost cheese; Olive oil;

Instead choose: Milk; Soybean oil; Yogurt;

Desserts, Snacks, Beverages

Sweet chocolate; Pound cake; Chocolate chip cookies; Chocolate ice cream; various cookies; Pie crust; Puff pastry; Dessert toppings; Cheesecake; Chocolate mousse; Coffeecake; Yellow cake; Coffee liqueur; Chocolate cake; Éclairs; various cakes; Cream puffs; Vanilla cream pie; various pies; After-dinner mints; Vanilla ice cream; Carob cadies; Peanut brittle; Pretzels; Coffee; various candies; Dark chocolate; Hot chocolate; Pudding; Frostings; Pancakes; 80+ proof distilled alc. bev.; Fruit punch; Lemonade; Whiskey; Soft (carbonated) drinks; Chewing gum; Jams & Preserves; Sherbet; Crème de menthe; Ice cream cones; Plain tea; Honey; Oil popped popcorn;

Instead choose: Taro chips; Peanut butter; Tonic water; Red wine; White wine; Potato chips/fried snacks; Sports drinks; Potato sticks; Applesauce; Ginger ale; Herbal tea; Eggnog; Malted (nonalcoholic) drinks; Beer;

Herbs & Spices, Fast Foods, Prepared Foods

Blue/Roquefort salad dressing; Foie gras or liver pate; French salad dressing; Mayonnaise; Hot dog; Cheese sauce; Table salt; Italian salad dressing; Oyster sauce; Nachos; Hoisin & Sofrito sauce; Pizza; Chocolate syrup; Barbecue sauce; Capers; Hash brown potatoes; Chicken Nuggets; Breaded shrimp; Cheeseburger; Table sugar (white or powder); Onion rings; Beef broth; Veg/beef soup; Taco shells; Ketchup; Tabasco sauce; Beef stock; Table blends syrup; Hush puppies; Pickle relish; Fish sauce; Maple syrup; Mustard; Potato salad; Hamburger; Pickle (cucumber); Gravies (canned); French toast; Macaroni; Tapioca; Potato pancakes; Cocoa; Maple sugar; Hummus; Sauerkraut; Vegetable soup; Croutons; Nutmeg; Chicken broth; Chicken noodle soup; Malt syrup; Corn cakes;

Instead choose: Chervil; French fries; Cinnamon; Cole slaw; Pepper (black or white); Turmeric; Cloves; Saffron; Fish stock; Mints; Poppy seed; Horseradish; Chicken stock; Mustard seed; Chives; Mace; Soy sauce; Ginger; Marjoram; Brown sugar; Vinegar; Clam chowder; Cardamom; Egg rolls (veg); Minestrone soup; Falafel; Sweet pickle;

Alternative Therapies & Miscellaneous

2+ alcoholic drinks/day; Excess body weight; Smoking, tobacco; Fried or battered foods; Hyperthermia (avoid if extremely high blood pressure); Stress; Salted foods, nuts, etc.; Corn sweetener; Sugared fruit juice or from concentrate; Birth control pills; Canned foods; Processed or Refined foods; Prescription drugs;

Key Nutrients & Herbal Medicines

Caffeine; Saturated fat; Total fat (limit to 30% of total daily calories); Licorice; Sodium/salt (limit to 1500 mg per day); Alcohol; Asian Ginseng; Refined sugar; Zinc (do not exceed RDA); Guarana; Kola (cola); Mate;

Cancer Risk (& HBP)

Cells are the building block of every organ in our body. Cells reproduce or die at varying rates depending on the organ and our age. Sometimes we have abnormal cells that reproduce or divide at a faster rate than we need. This phenomenon results in a collection of unwanted cells called a tumor. If the cells in the tumor have the ability to infiltrate other tissues and organs in our body then this tumor is considered malignant, otherwise it is considered benign. Cancer is the condition that corresponds to the malignant tumors. Cancer refers to as many as 200 different diseases but they all have the out of control cell reproduction in common.

Cancers are named after the organ where a tumor first appears. Some cancers do not form a tumor such as cancer of blood. In medical jargon, if cancer affects soft tissues and organs such as breast or lung, they are categorized as Carcinomas. If cancer affects hard tissues such as bone or muscle, they are called Sarcomas. If cancer affects our lymphatic system (i.e., part of body's circulatory system which transports things such as plasma, fats, white cells from one place to another throughout our body), it is called Lymphoma. And finally if cancer affects tissues such as blood or bone marrow, it is known as Leukemia.

There has been significant progress in cancer research and treatment of cancer over the recent decades. We understand that gene mutations are the cause of cancer development. We also know of most of the causes for gene mutations that cause cancer, i.e., the carcinogens. In short, the research has led to identification of various risk factors that increase the possibility of developing cancer. The most common of which are: family history of cancer; age (growing older); exposure to Ultraviolet (UV) radiation (from sun, tanning booths, sunlamps); certain infections; hormones (e.g., estrogen); exposure to certain chemicals (e.g., radon gas, asbestos); alcohol; tobacco; poor diet; stress; obesity and lack of physical activity. Having several risk factors does NOT mean that one will get cancer. Conversely, absence of risk factors does not mean that one will not get cancer.

The suggestions and information presented in this book are primarily focused on prevention of various cancer types through avoidance of the known risk factors for the specific cancer type. When known, information about food items or actions that could shrink or slow down growth of tumors is included. It is important to note that, there is no definitive cure, treatment or preventive measure that is known and certain for any specific type of cancer at this time.

Few words on phytochemicals, antioxidants, free radicals ...

Phytochemicals are substances or compounds found in many plants. They are also known by other names among them antioxidants and flavonoids. While thousands of phytochemicals have been discovered, very few have been studied in detail. Some of the better known phytochemicals (antioxidants) are beta carotene, Vitamin C, folic acid and Vitamin E.

Various studies and many experts suggest that the risk of cancer can be significantly reduced by eating more fruits, vegetables, beans and whole grains that contain phytochemicals. There is some evidence that certain phytochemicals may prevent formation of tumors, or suppress cancer development. But there is no data that supports taking phytochemical supplements is as effective as consuming fruits, vegetables, beans and grains as part of a normal diet. Nor are supplements regulated by the FDA. Thus, taking phytochemicals in form of supplements is not recommended.

One group of these compounds, known as antioxidants, may protect our cells against free radicals. Free radicals are molecules produced by our body as it breaks down food or by exposure to things such as tobacco smoke or radiation. Free radicals can damage our cell's DNA and are linked to certain diseases including cancer. Antioxidants are thought to eliminate free radicals, and slow down oxidation, which is a natural process that leads to damage to the cells and tissue in our body.

Another group of these compounds is known as flavonoids. Some studies suggest that some of these compounds may protect against hormone-dependent cancers such as breast and prostate cancers. Another group of flavonoids act as antioxidants, and thus have protective and anti-cancer properties.

A third group of Phytochemicals, called Allyl Sulfides, may help our body get rid of harmful chemicals and strengthen our immune system.

Many of the dietary recommendations that you find in this chapter are based on the various known phytochemical content and their effect on various types of cancer.

Choose these for High Blood Pressure & Cancer Risk

Top 5 items to consume:

Garlic; Dried Fruits; Soymilk/Soybeans; Green leafy vegetables; Mushrooms;

Food items and actions that could improve your health or reduce your risk (within a food group, the most helpful items are listed first):

Meat, Fish & Poultry

Fish roe; Pink salmon; White fish; Mackerel; Snail; Trout; Ling; Sturgeon; Herring; Seabass; Snapper; Spot; Pompano fish; Blue fin tuna; Sardines; Pollock; Pout; Smelt; Whiting; Catfish; Marlin; Wolffish; Eel; Carp; Whelk; Yellowtail; Monkfish; Scup; Swordfish; Freshwater bass; Walleye; Spiny lobster; Lingcod; Chicken liver & giblet; Octopus; Halibut; Turkey liver; Mullet; Shad; Mussels; Striped bass; Tilapia; Cusk; Sucker; Sheepshead; Caviar; Dolphinfish (Mahi-Mahi); Crayfish; Drum; Turkey giblets; Dungeness crab; Milkfish; Turbot; Blue crab; Bluefish; Surimi; Rockfish; Calamari; Perch; Pumpkinseed sunfish; Oysters; Burbot; Cisco (smoked); Northern pike; Cisco; Flatfish (flounder & sole); Beef liver; Tilefish; Butterfish; Anchovy; Pork liver;

Eggs, Beans, Nuts and Seeds

Split peas; Breadnut tree seeds; Soy milk; Soybeans (green); Beans: adzuki, navy, moth beans, winged, hyacinth, black, pinto; Chickpeas; Lentils; various beans; Chia seeds; Ginkgo nuts; Flaxseed[1]; Sunflower seeds; Green peas; Black-eyed peas; Alfalfa sprouts; Hazelnuts or Filberts; Sugar or snap peas; Breadfruit seeds; Lupin; Almonds; Walnuts; Soybean seeds; Chestnuts; Cottonseed; Peanuts; Brazil nuts; Safflower seeds; Pistachio nuts; Pine nuts; Beechnuts; Black walnuts; Acorns; Watermelon seeds; Sesame seeds; Butternuts; Cashew nuts; Coconut meat (dried); Pili nuts; Pecans; Egg yolk; Hickory nuts; Cornnuts; Pumpkin & squash seeds;

Fruits & Juices *(Five servings of fruits & Veg daily. Avoid non-organic. Wash fruits & vegetables well and peel their skin)*

Dried: Banana, Litchi, Prunes, Peaches, Apricots, Currants; Tamarind; Goji berry; Passion fruit; other dried fruits; Raisins; Guava; Plantains; Abiyuch; Elderberries; Currants (raw); Dates; Kiwi fruit; Apricots; Blackberries; Boysenberries; Cantaloupe; Kumquats; Persimmons; various berries; Rowal; Cranberry juice; Lemon; Peaches; Breadfruit; Pineapple juice; Orange juice; Banana; Grapefruit; Mango; Oranges; Papaya; Plum; Jujube (fruit); Longans; Acerola; Pumelo (Shaddock); Lime; Watermelon; Durian; Natal Plum (Carissa); Pitanga; Tangerines; Grapefruit juice; Nectarine; Avocado; Apples; Pineapple; Prune juice; Figs; Pomegranate; Grape juice; Grapes; Pears; Rhubarb; Cherries; Cranberries; Apple juice; Quince; Honeydew melon; Pomegranate juice; Strawberries; Olives;

Vegetables *(Five servings of fruits & Veg daily. Avoid non-organic. Wash fruits & vegetables well and peel their skin)*

Garlic (take raw or crushed but not heated immediately); Amaranth leaves; Epazote; Fungi cloud ears; Grape leaves; Shitake mushrooms; Ancho and pasilla peppers; Pigeon peas; Sun-dried tomatoes; Wasabi root; Taro leaves; Balsam pear leafy tips; Sweet potatoes leaves; Tahitian taro; Vine spinach (Basella); Artichoke; Chrysanthemum (Garland); Chrysanthemum Leaves; Dandelion Greens; Mustard spinach; Garden cress; Kale; Arugula; Chinese broccoli; Chicory greens; Collards; Mustard greens; Okra; Turnip greens; Bok choy; Borage; Cowpeas leafy tips; Purslane; Watercress; Winged beans leaves; Arrowhead; Cauliflower; Beet greens; Broccoli; Brussels sprouts; Endive; Green onions (scallions); Kohlrabi; Taro; Kelp; Nopal; Celtuce; Hot chili peppers; Rutabaga; Spinach; Winter squash; Yam; various cabbage; Green beans; various peppers; Parsnips; Arrowroot; Lambsquarters; Bell peppers; various lettuce; Pokeberry shoots; Pumpkin; Pumpkin flowers; Radishes; Sesbania Flower; Lotus root; Potatoes w/skin; Turnips; Swiss chard; Onions (2-5 oz. of fresh onion daily, or 1 tsp. onion juice 3-4 times a day); other vegetables;

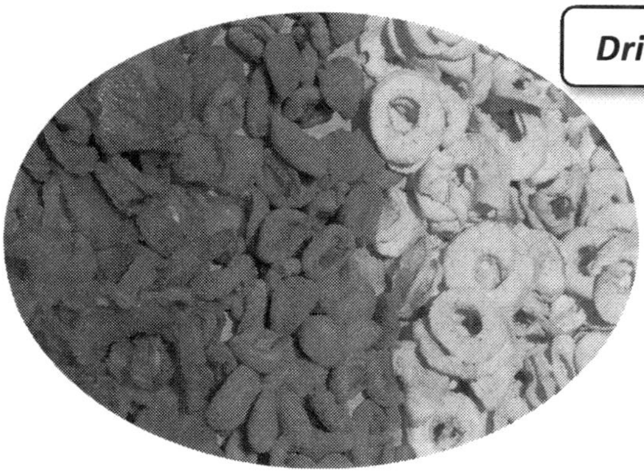

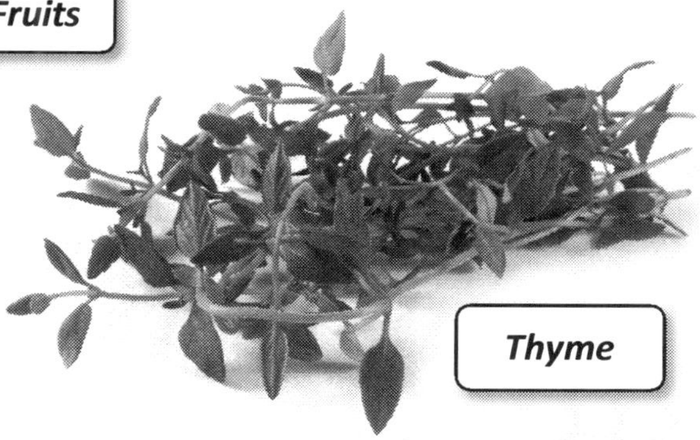

Breads, Grains, Cereals, Pasta

Rye; Corn bran; Buckwheat; Oats; Amaranth; Triticale; Sorghum; Rice bran; Bran flakes cereal; Oatmeal (cereal); Barley; Corn; Millet; Brown rice; Wild rice; Oat bran muffins; Rice cakes (Brown rice based); Tortillas (corn); Granola cereal; Durum wheat; Wheat germ cereal; Whole-wheat bread; Spelt (cooked); Whole-wheat English muffins; Bulgur; Whole-wheat cereal; Whole-wheat spaghetti; Whole-wheat dinner rolls; Wheat germ bread; Shredded wheat; Wheat bran muffins; Wheat bran; Wheat germ; Whole-wheat;

Dairy Products, Fats & Oils

Whey (dried); Cod Liver Fish Oil; Wheat Germ Oil; Gjetost cheese; Yogurt; various fish oil; Fat-free or Low Fat products

Desserts, Snacks, Beverages

Air-popped Popcorn; Blackstrap molasses; Red wine; Water (pure water, not tap water); Sesame crunch candies; Molasses; Green tea (do not brew or drink boiling hot); White wine;

Herbs & Spices, Fast Foods, Prepared Foods

Thyme (fresh); Tofu; Peppermint; Whole-grain cornmeal; Parsley; Fried tofu; Dill weed; Spearmint (fresh); Coriander/Cilantro; Tempeh; Cottonseed meal; Natto; Rosemary (fresh); Minestrone soup; Cocoa; Corn salad; Egg rolls (veg); Vegetable soup; Oregano; Sage; Cayenne (red) pepper; Basil (fresh); Cheese fondue; Tomato paste; Succotash; Tarragon (dried); Pepper (black or white); Turmeric; French fries; Mints; Chervil; Maple sugar; Mace; Fennel seeds; Sorghum syrup; Cole slaw; Marjoram; Poppy seed; Cinnamon; Nutmeg; Chives;

Alternative Therapies & Miscellaneous

Consult your doctor (ask for screening); Exercise; Organically grown foods (Avoid non-organic foods. If not possible, wash fruits/vegs well and peel off their skin); Follow DASH diet; Fresh (uncooked) fruits/veg's or use no salt added canned; Fat-free or low fat products; Salt-free or low-salt foods; Wild fish and free range animals (avoid animals raised on antibiotics or grains); Anti-inflammation diet; Meditation; Ornish Plan & Diet; Pray, practice your religion; Sleep 6-8 hours regularly; Tai Chi; Vegetarian diet; Yoga (avoid certain postures);

Key Nutrients & Herbal Medicines

Fiber; Hawthorn (in berries form or tea from dried leaves and flowers. Do not take with other heart medications); Beta Carotene (do not take in supplement form); Bugleweed; Calcium; Celery seed; Foxglove; Siberian Ginseng; Magnesium; Omega-3 fatty acids (to prevent breast, prostate and colon cancers in particular); Potassium; Vitamin D; Yucca;

Do not choose these for High Blood Pressure & Cancer Risk

Top 5 items to avoid:

Cured & Luncheon (processed) Meats; Sweets; Salad dressings & Sauces; Smoking & Alcohol; Hydrogenated Vegetable Oil

Avoid or consume much less of the following (within a food group, most harmful items are listed first):

Meat, Fish & Poultry

Chorizo; Frankfurters; Luncheon meats; Pepperoni; Pork skins; Salami; various sausage; Bacon; Pork liver cheese; Cured beef; Pastrami; Beef jerky sticks; Bologna; Meatless sausage; Pork cured/ham; Corned beef; Cured meats; Turkey skins; Beef tongue; Pork headcheese; Beef ribs; Lamb tongue; Salmon (smoked, Lox); Beef chuck/brisket; Pork ribs; Lamb ribs; Pork spare ribs; Chicken skin; Ground beef; Beef; Lamb; Pork; Meat (limit consumption of red meat; choose organic); Bison/buffalo meat; Squab (pigeon); Veal tongue; Veal; Rabbit meat; Venison; Organ meats; Goose; Chicken dark meat; Quail; Boar meat; White fish (smoked); Beef filet mignon; Chicken wings; Orange roughy;

Instead choose: King mackerel; Seatrout; Cod; Yellowfin tuna; Cuttlefish; Alaskan King crab; Chicken breast (no skin); Haddock; Abalone; Shark; Turkey; Veal liver; Grouper; Shrimp; Clams; Canned tuna;

Eggs, Beans, Nuts and Seeds

Coconut Milk;

Instead choose: Macadamia nuts; Coconut; Egg; Egg white; Egg substitute;

Breads, Grains, Cereals, Pasta

Saltines crackers; Danish pastry; Croissant; Milk crackers; Wheat crackers; Donuts; Sweet rolls; Granola bars; French rolls; White bread; Biscuits; Rice crisps cereal; Kaiser dinner rolls; Hamburger & hot dog rolls; Melba toasts crackers; Wheat; Bagels; Matzo crackers; Blueberry muffins; Bread sticks; Banana bread; Cream of wheat cereal; Corn flakes; Cornbread;

Instead choose: Spinach spaghetti; Oat bran; Semolina; Egg noodles; Couscous; Spaghetti; White rice; Whole-wheat crackers; Corn muffins; Pumpernickel bread;

Dairy Products, Fats & Oils

Hydrogenated vegetable oil; Vegetable shortening; Butter (salted); American cheese; Margarine; Margarine-like spreads; Animal fat; Oils: Cupu Assu, sesame, Shea nut, tea seed, Ucuhuba Butter; Pimento cheese; Butter (unsalted); various cheese; Cocoa Butter oil; Avocado oil; Lard; Poultry fats; Cheese spread; Chocolate milk; various veg's/seeds/nuts oils; Whipped cream; Cream; Sour cream; Canola oil; Gruyere cheese;

Instead choose: Cottage cheese; Flaxseed oil; Swiss cheese; Milk; Ricotta cheese;

Desserts, Snacks, Beverages

Pound cake; Cookies: butter, chocolate chip, shortbread; Puff pastry; various cookies; Chocolate cake; Éclairs; various cakes; Cream puffs; Pretzels; Pie crust; Chocolate ice cream; Sweet chocolate; Cheesecake; Pudding; Dessert toppings; Coffeecake; various types of pie; Chocolate mousse; Fruit leather/rolls; After-dinner mints; Soft (carbonated) drinks; Honey; Coffee liqueur; Vanilla ice cream; Peanut brittle candies; Pancakes; Coffee; Ice cream cones; Lemonade; various candies; Frostings; Tortilla chips; Fruit punch; Potato sticks; Hot chocolate; Chewing gum; Sherbet; Hard candies; Frozen yogurt; Jams & Preserves; Taro chips; 80+ proof distilled alcoholic beverages;

Instead choose: Dark chocolate; Peanut butter; Plain tea; Pumpkin pie; Herbal tea; Milk shakes; Malted drinks (non-alcoholic); Beer; Piña colada; Eggnog;

Herbs & Spices, Fast Foods, Prepared Foods

Blue/Roquefort & French salad dressings; Oyster sauce; Italian salad dressing; Sofrito & Hoisin sauces; Hot dog; Barbecue sauce; various sauces; Breaded shrimp; Chicken Nuggets; Table sugar (white or powder); Nachos; Pizza; Table salt; Mayonnaise; Hush puppies; Ketchup; Onion rings; Cheeseburger; Tabasco sauce; Foie gras or liver pate; Capers; Tapioca; Macaroni; Chocolate syrup; Hamburger; Pickle relish; Syrup (table blends); Pickle (cucumber); Beef broth; Soy sauce; Hash brown potatoes; Gravies (canned); Taco shells; various syrup; Mustard; Beef stock; Potato salad; Chicken noodle soup; Hummus; French toast;

Instead choose: Cardamom; Horseradish; Miso; Ginger; Saffron; Fish stock; Cloves; Mustard seed; Falafel; Tomato soup; Brown sugar; Veg/beef soup; Croutons; Chicken stock; Vinegar; Teriyaki sauce; Potato pancakes;

Alternative Therapies & Miscellaneous

2+ alcoholic drinks/day; Smoking, tobacco; Excess body weight; Processed or Refined foods (avoid any and all manufactured foods); Stress; Pesticide-loaded crops; Salted foods, nuts, etc.; Corn sweetener; Sugared fruit juice or from concentrate; Air pollutants; Food additives Nitrates/Nitrites; Smoked foods; Harsh chemicals & fumes; Hyperthermia (avoid if extremely high blood pressure); Non-organic foods; Radiation (from X-rays, television, microwave, computer, cell phones); Fried or battered foods;

Key Nutrients & Herbal Medicines

Sodium/salt (limit to 1500 mg per day); Caffeine; Betel Nut; Total fat; Licorice; Mercury (avoid heavy metal loaded fish); Refined sugar; Trans fatty acids; Saturated fat; Guarana; Kola (cola); Mate;

Stress (& HBP)

Everyone experiences some sort of stress almost every day. Stress is our brain's response to a demand. Not everyone reacts to the same events or demands the same way. What may be stressful to one person may not be to another. It is stress that drives us to act, and in some cases such as survival situations, perform beyond our normal abilities. However, long term or chronic stress can lead to a variety of problems including illnesses such as high blood pressure, depression and cancer.

Chronic stress can be caused by a number of factors, among them: bad childhood experiences (whose pain and impact you have never been able to escape), poverty and helplessness, an unhappy marriage, never-ending tension and violence all around you, a wrong job or career, and a dysfunctional family.

Chronic stress challenges our mind and body over a long time, and thus may require an on-going treatment over an extended period of time.

Choose these for High Blood Pressure & Stress

Top 5 items to consume:

Garlic; Dark Green Leafy Vegetables; Seeds & Ginkgo nuts; Wheat Bran/Germ; Salmon;

Food items and actions that could improve your health (within a food group, most helpful items are listed first):

Meat, Fish & Poultry

Pink salmon; Marlin; Swordfish; Whelk; Yellowfin tuna; Snapper; Fish roe; Mackerel; Blue fin tuna; Spot; Halibut; White fish; Trout; Bluefish; King mackerel; Octopus; Carp; Pollock; Herring; Tilefish; Sardines; Sturgeon; Wolffish; Beef liver; Veal thymus; Milkfish; Striped bass; Snail; Beef spleen; Caviar; Catfish; Ling; Drum; Seabass; Cusk; Sheepshead; Chicken liver; Freshwater bass; Perch; Walleye; Lingcod; Scup; Smelt; Shark; Whiting; Veal spleen; Monkfish; Liver; Sucker; Cisco (smoked); Pout; Yellowtail; Pompano fish; Dolphinfish (Mahi-Mahi); Pumpkinseed sunfish; Burbot; Northern pike; Shad; Tilapia; Beef filet mignon; Butterfish; Mullet; Seatrout; Rockfish; Cisco; Surimi; Spiny lobster; Eel; Turbot; Haddock; Mussels; Grouper; Cuttlefish; Sablefish; Dungeness crab; White fish (smoked); Chicken breast (no skin); Crayfish; Rabbit meat; Blue crab; Pheasant; Beef/lamb brain; Flatfish (flounder & sole); Pork loin/sirloin; Beef rib eye; Beef; Canned tuna; Pheasant breast; Calamari; Clams; Oysters; Veal shank; Cod; Veal; Croaker; Turkey breast; Scallops; Alaskan King crab; Anchovy; Lamb leg; Boar meat; Shrimp; Quail breast; Bison/buffalo meat; Turkey dark meat; Quail; Orange roughy; Pork leg/ham; Lamb shoulder;

Eggs, Beans, Nuts and Seeds

Breadnut tree seeds; Ginkgo nuts; Seeds: safflower, sunflower, cottonseed; Sugar or snap peas; Pistachio nuts; Hazelnuts or Filberts; Flaxseed; Green peas; Soy milk; Chestnuts; Butternuts; Black walnuts; Soybean seeds; Soybeans (green); Almonds; Walnuts; Breadfruit seeds; Split peas; Beechnuts; Chia seeds; Pine nuts; Brazil nuts; Watermelon seeds; Pili nuts; Pumpkin & squash seeds; Cashew nuts; Sesame seeds; Pinto beans; Lentils; Peanuts; Acorns; various beans; Chickpeas; Hickory nuts; Black-eyed peas; Alfalfa sprouts; Lupin; Pecans; Egg yolk; Cornnuts; Macadamia nuts; Egg; Coconut meat (dried);

Fruits & Juices

Dried Litchi & Banana; Abiyuch; Guava; Pineapple juice; Currants; Kiwi fruit; Goji berry; Jujube (fruit); Longans; Persimmons; Prunes (dried); Raisins; Orange juice; Lemon; Elderberries; Tamarind; Dates; Acerola; Litchi; Oranges; Papaya; Pumelo (Shaddock); Strawberries; dried figs; Kumquats; dried peaches, Longans, Apricots; Banana; Passion fruit; Pineapple; Prune juice; Cantaloupe; Natal Plum (Carissa); Grapefruit juice; dried fruits; Mango; various berries; Breadfruit; Avocado; Grape juice; Plantains; Cranberry juice; Durian; Lime; Pears; Apricots; Grapefruit; Apple juice; Figs; Pomegranate; Rowal; Apples; Grapes; Peaches; Cherries; Nectarine; Plum; Pomegranate juice; Watermelon; Pitanga; Tangerines; Honeydew melon; Quince; Rhubarb; Cranberries; Olives;

Vegetables

Garlic; Sun-dried tomatoes; Amaranth leaves; Taro leaves; Wasabi root; Balsam pear leafy tips; Tahitian taro; Vine spinach (Basella); Mustard spinach; Garden cress; Kale; Mustard greens; Turnip greens; Shitake mushrooms; Ancho & pasilla peppers; Dandelion Greens; Bok choy; Winged beans leaves; Balsam pear; Broccoli; Brussels sprouts; Kohlrabi; Cauliflower; Hot chili peppers; Collards; Watercress; Lambsquarters; various peppers; Cowpeas leafy tips; Bell peppers; Red cabbage; Pokeberry shoots; Sesbania Flower; Borage; Grape leaves; Chinese broccoli; Spinach; Okra; Pigeon peas; Green cabbage; Beet greens; Epazote; Fungi cloud ears; Savoy cabbage; Lotus root; Arrowhead; Chicory greens; Sweet potatoes leaves; Purslane; Potatoes w/skin; Arugula; Pumpkin flowers; Chrysanthemum (Garland); Chrysanthemum Leaves; Rutabaga; Swiss chard; Artichoke; Taro; Yellow squash; Zucchini; Yam; Shallots; Kelp; Nopal; Parsnips; Fiddlehead ferns; Green onions (scallions); Celtuce; Potato; Arrowroot; Portabella mushrooms; Quinoa seed; Winter squash; Onions (2-5 oz. of fresh onion daily, or 1 tsp. onion juice 3-4 times a day); Carrots; Endive; Radishes; other vegetables;

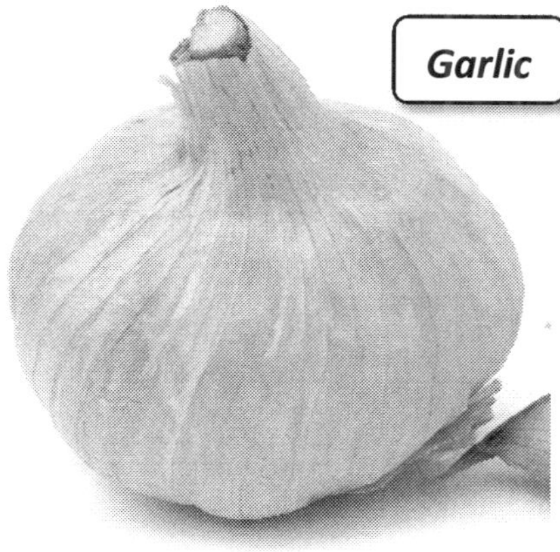

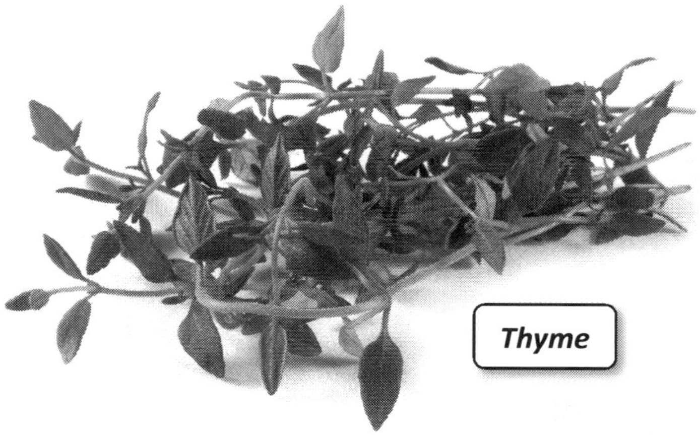

Breads, Grains, Cereals, Pasta

Wheat bran; Wheat germ; Wheat germ cereal; Bran flakes cereal; Rice bran; Wheat bran muffins; Wheat germ bread; Amaranth; Whole-wheat; Durum wheat; Buckwheat; Shredded wheat cereal; Whole-wheat bread; Rye; Oats; Whole-wheat spaghetti; Whole-wheat English muffins; Corn bran; Whole-wheat cereal; Triticale; Oatmeal (cereal); Oat bran muffins; Corn flakes; Sorghum; Brown rice; Spelt (cooked); Whole-wheat dinner rolls; Millet; Granola cereal; Barley; Bulgur; Rice cakes (Brown rice based); Rice crisps cereal; Corn; Wild rice; Tortillas (corn); Whole-wheat crackers; Oat bran bread; Oat bran; Semolina; Pumpernickel bread; Spinach spaghetti; White rice;

Dairy Products, Fats & Oils

Whey (dried); Wheat Germ Oil; Cheeses: Gjetost, Swiss, Gruyere, cottage; Cod Liver Fish Oil; Flaxseed Oil; Port de salut cheese; Fish oils: Herring, salmon, sardine; Mozzarella cheese; Milk, 2% fat; Fat-free or Low Fat products; Salt-free or Low Salt products.

Desserts, Snacks, Beverages

Molasses; Sesame crunch candies; Air-popped popcorn; Potato chips/fried snacks; Peanut butter; Potato sticks; Fruit leather/rolls; Halvah; Water;

Herbs & Spices, Fast Foods, Prepared Foods

Thyme (fresh); Cottonseed meal; Parsley; Dill weed; Peppermint; Rosemary (fresh); Whole-grain cornmeal; Tofu; Sorghum syrup; Corn salad; Cheese fondue; Natto; Coriander/Cilantro; Tomato paste; Tempeh; Basil (fresh); Tarragon (dried); Spearmint (fresh); Potato pancakes; French fries; Cole slaw; Pepper or hot sauce; Cayenne (red) pepper; Oregano; Sage; Chervil; Clam chowder; Succotash; Malt syrup; Fennel seeds; Pepper (black or white); Turmeric;

Alternative Therapies & Miscellaneous

Exercise regularly; Meditation; Sleep 6-8 hours regularly; Yoga (avoid certain positions); Follow DASH diet; Fresh (uncooked) fruits/veg's or no salt added canned; Laugh, laughter; Pray, practice your religion; Tai Chi; Biofeedback; Fat-free or low fat products; Hypnotherapy; Ornish Plan & Diet; Sexual activity; Sound Therapy; Take a vacation!; Salt-free or low-salt foods; Organically grown foods;

Key Nutrients & Herbal Medicines

Siberian Ginseng; Hawthorn (in berries form or tea from dried leaves and flowers; do not take with other heart medications); Vitamin C (Ascorbic acid); Magnesium; Ashwaganda; Calcium; Celery seed; Potassium; Vitamin B-6; Yucca;

<u>Do not</u> choose these for High Blood Pressure & Stress

Top 5 items to avoid:

Chocolate & Sweets; 2+ Alcoholic drinks/day; Caffeine & Smoking; Margarine & Hydrogenated vegetable oil ... & Excess body weight;

Avoid or consume much less of the following (within a food group, most harmful items are listed first):

Meat, Fish & Poultry

Pork skins; Cured meats; Sausage; Pastrami; Frankfurters; Beerwurst beer salami; Luncheon meats; Chicken skin; Bacon; Pepperoni; Pork breakfast strips; Beef jerky sticks; Cured beef; Chorizo; Pork liver cheese;

Instead <u>choose</u>: Guinea hen; Venison; Lobster; Abalone; Lamb loin; Ground lamb; Pork; Duck (no skin); Beef shank; Lamb ribs; Lamb tongue; Beef ribs; Goose; Chicken dark meat; Chicken wings; Salmon (smoked, lox); Beef chuck/brisket; Meatless sausage;

Eggs, Beans, Nuts and Seeds

Coconut Milk;

Instead <u>choose</u>: Egg (raw); Egg substitute; Coconut; Egg white;

Breads, Grains, Cereals, Pasta

Saltines crackers; Croissant; Danish Pastry; Sweet rolls; Milk crackers; Kaiser dinner rolls; French rolls; Wheat crackers; Donuts; Biscuits; White Bread; Chinese chow Mein noodles;

Instead <u>choose</u>: Wheat; Corn muffins; Cornbread; Banana bread; Cream of wheat; Egg noodles; Couscous; Japanese noodles; Rice noodles; Pasta; Spaghetti; Italian bread;

Dairy Products, Fats & Oils

Margarine (salted); Margarine-like spreads; Hydrogenated vegetable oil; Margarine (unsalted); Animal fat; Oils: Babassu, Cocoa Butter, cottonseed, Cupu Assu, palm, peanut, poppy seed, rice bran, sesame, Shea nut, tea seed, Ucuhuba Butter; Chocolate milk; Butter (salted); Lard; various veg's/seeds/nuts oils; Vegetable shortening; Poultry fats; Butter (unsalted); Goat cheese; Whipped cream; Cheeses: Roquefort, pimento, cream, Brie; Canola oil;

Instead <u>choose</u>: Menhaden fish oil; Gouda cheese; Milk; Cheeses: Cheddar, Colby, Edam; Yogurt; Ricotta & Fontina cheeses; other cheese;

Desserts, Snacks, Beverages

Sweet chocolate; Chocolate ice cream; Coffee liqueur; Chocolate chip cookies; Shortbread cookies; Pie crust; Puff pastry; Pound cake; various cookies; Chocolate cake; Coffee; Cheesecake; various cakes; Éclairs; Pretzels; Dessert toppings; Cream puffs; Coffeecake; Hot chocolate; Chocolate mousse; various pies; After-dinner mints; Plain tea; Peanut brittle candies; Vanilla ice cream; Soft (carbonated) drinks; Ice cream cones; Frostings; Pudding; Fruit punch; Lemonade; Pancakes; Pumpkin pie; Honey; 80+ proof distilled alc. bev.; Whiskey;

Instead choose: Tortilla chips; Taro chips; Milk shakes; Tonic water; Red wine; White wine; Eggnog; Malted drinks (non-alcoholic); Sports drinks; Dark chocolate; Applesauce; Ginger ale; Herbal tea; Beer; Frozen yogurt; Peanut bar candies;

Herbs & Spices, Fast Foods, Prepared Foods

Salad dressings: Blue/Roquefort, French; Table salt; Italian salad dressing; Sauces: oyster, Hoisin, barbecue; Capers; Mayonnaise; Cheese sauce; Chocolate syrup; Table sugar (white or powder); Breaded shrimp; Hot dog; Foie gras or liver pate; Onion rings; Soy sauce; Chicken Nuggets; Ketchup; Tabasco sauce; Syrup (table blends); Pickle relish; Pizza; Pickle (cucumber); Hash brown potatoes; Mustard; Sofrito sauce; Gravies (canned);

Instead choose: Miso; Poppy seed; Horseradish; Fish stock; Saffron; Falafel; Chives; Cinnamon; Mustard seed; Hamburger; Mints; Maple sugar; Cocoa; Beef stock; Chicken stock; Hummus; Cardamom; Mace; Teriyaki sauce; Taco shells; Cloves; Fish sauce; Ginger; Marjoram; Brown sugar; Vinegar; Nutmeg; Minestrone soup; Sauerkraut; Beef broth; Chicken broth; Chicken noodle soup; Veg/beef soup;

Alternative Therapies & Miscellaneous

2+ alcoholic drinks/day; Excess body weight; Smoking, tobacco; Hyperthermia (avoid if extremely high blood pressure); Stress; Birth control pills; Salted foods, nuts, etc.; FD&C yellow dye #5. Tartrazine; Corn sweetener; Sugared fruit juice or from concentrate;

Key Nutrients & Herbal Medicines

Caffeine; Licorice; Sodium (salt); Guarana; Kola (cola); Mate;

Vitamin D Deficiency (& HBP)

Vitamin D Deficiency is a common problem for many people especially the older people. Vitamin D is a critical nutrient for your body in particular for stronger bones, muscle movements, nerve function and immune system well-being.

You will develop this deficiency if you don't absorb enough Vitamin D from your diet, you don't get enough exposure to the sun (especially during the winter months), your skin cannot convert the sun exposure to Vitamin D (as in elderly and darker skin), or you are obese. You can also develop this deficiency if your body cannot properly process fats due to Celiac or Crohn's disease, since fats are required for Vitamin D absorption into your blood. Health issues with kidney and liver can also result in this deficiency because they can prevent your body to process Vitamin D.

Adults, ages 19 to 70, require 600 IU (International Units) of Vitamin D per day. Adults, ages 71 and above, require 800 IU per day.

Meeting your Vitamin D needs entirely through sun exposure or tanning is not recommended due to the risk of skin cancer. Too much Vitamin D in your blood (almost always caused by supplements) can also be harmful.

Choose these for High Blood Pressure & Vitamin D Deficiency

Top 5 items to choose:

**Fish & Fish oil; Almonds & Hazelnuts;
Prunes & Raisins; Soybeans;
Beans/Legumes; & get some Sun!**

Food items and actions that could improve your health (within a food group, most helpful items are listed first):

Meat, Fish & Poultry

Pink salmon; Fish roe; Marlin; Swordfish; White fish; Trout; Snapper; Carp; Mackerel; Sturgeon; Catfish; Pompano fish; Cisco (smoked); Eel; Blue fin tuna; Seabass; Herring; Halibut; White fish (smoked); Sardines; Perch; Snail; Walleye; Shad; Caviar; Whelk; Tilapia; Whiting; Ling; Rockfish; Yellowfin tuna; Spot; Monkfish; Tilefish; Pollock; Freshwater bass; Mullet; Pout; Bluefish; King mackerel; Smelt; Northern pike; Flatfish (flounder & sole); Striped bass; Yellowtail; Drum; Sucker; Wolffish; Sheepshead; Lingcod; Scup; Octopus; Milkfish; Burbot; Cusk; Pumpkinseed sunfish; Shark; Dolphinfish (Mahi-Mahi); Mussels; Grouper; Surimi; Cisco; Spiny lobster; Crayfish; Turbot; Anchovy; Calamari; Pork loin/sirloin; Butterfish; Seatrout;

Eggs, Beans, Nuts and Seeds

Almonds; Hazelnuts or Filberts; Soybean seeds; Split peas; Soybeans (green); Beans: adzuki, navy, moth beans, winged; Seeds: breadnut tree, chia, cottonseed, flaxseed, safflower; Soy milk; various beans; Sunflower seeds; Chickpeas; Lentils; Breadfruit seeds; Pine nuts; Pistachio nuts; Brazil nuts; Peanuts; Watermelon seeds; Ginkgo nuts; Butternuts; Black walnuts; Pili nuts; Pumpkin & squash seeds; Walnuts; Green peas; Black-eyed peas; Alfalfa sprouts; Cashew nuts; Lupin; Sugar or snap peas; Chestnuts; Pecans; Beechnuts; Hickory nuts; Acorns; Egg yolk; Sesame seeds; Cornnuts;

Fruits & Juices

Prunes (dried); Raisins; Dried Banana & Litchi; Tamarind; dried Figs, Peaches, Apricots, Currants; Dates; Goji berry; dried Longans; Passion fruit; Grape juice; other dried fruits; Banana; Prune juice; Avocado; Abiyuch; Elderberries; Guava; Pineapple juice; Plantains; Pears; Cranberry juice; Breadfruit; Currants (raw); Durian; Kiwi fruit; Apricots; various berries; Cantaloupe; Jujube (fruit); Kumquats; Longans; Natal Plum (Carissa); Persimmons; Rowal; Apple juice; Grapefruit juice; Orange juice; Apples; Grapes; Peaches; Figs; Lemon; Lime; Pomegranate; Acerola; Cherries; Grapefruit; Honeydew melon; Litchi; Mango; Nectarine; Oranges; Papaya; Pineapple; Pitanga; Plum; Pomegranate juice; Pumelo (Shaddock); Quince; Strawberries; Tangerines; Watermelon;

Vegetables

Shitake mushrooms; Garlic; Amaranth leaves; Epazote; Fungi cloud ears; Grape leaves; Ancho & pasilla peppers; Pigeon peas; Sun-dried tomatoes; Wasabi root; Taro leaves; Arrowhead; Balsam pear leafy tips; Sweet potatoes leaves; Tahitian taro; Vine spinach (Basella); Artichoke; Chrysanthemum (Garland); Chrysanthemum Leaves; Dandelion Greens; Mustard spinach; Garden cress; Kale; Arugula; Kelp; Nopal; Potatoes w/skin; Taro; Chinese broccoli; Chicory greens; Collards; Mustard greens; Okra; Turnip greens; Yam; Cauliflower; Bok choy; Borage; Cowpeas leafy tips; Purslane; Watercress; Winged beans leaves; Quinoa seed; Onions (2-5 oz. of fresh onion daily, or 1 tsp. onion juice 3-4 times a day); Lotus root; Parsnips; Beet greens; Balsam pear; Broccoli; Brussels sprouts; Carrots; Endive; Fiddlehead ferns; Green onions (scallions); Kohlrabi; Shallots; Arrowroot; Jerusalem artichoke; Portabella mushrooms; Beets; Celtuce; Hot chili peppers; Rutabaga; Spinach; Squash; Zucchini; Potato; Lambsquarters; Green & Savoy cabbage; Eggplant; Green beans; Banana & jalapeno peppers; other vegetables;

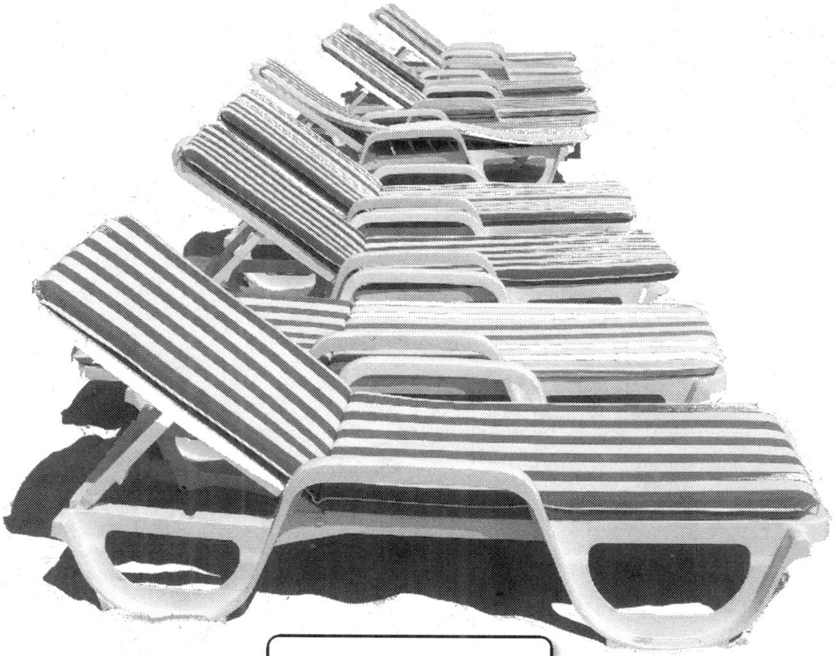

Get some sun!

Breads, Grains, Cereals, Pasta

Bran flakes cereal; Wheat bran; Wheat germ; Whole-wheat; Amaranth; Whole-wheat bread; Buckwheat; Wheat germ cereal; Durum wheat; Oats; Rye; Whole-wheat English muffins; Corn bran; Triticale; Whole-wheat cereal; Whole-wheat spaghetti; Rice bran; Sorghum; Oatmeal (cereal); Wheat bran muffins; Wheat germ bread; Spelt (cooked); Oat bran muffins; Millet; Brown rice; Barley; Bulgur; Whole-wheat dinner rolls; Shredded wheat cereal; Corn; Wild rice; Granola cereal; Rice cakes (Brown rice based); Tortillas (corn); Whole-wheat crackers;

Dairy Products, Fats & Oils

Cod liver fish oil; Whey (dried); Wheat germ oil; Sardine fish oil; Gjetost cheese; Cottage cheese; Flaxseed oil; Fish oils: herring, salmon; Swiss cheese;

Desserts, Snacks, Beverages

Sesame crunch candies; Molasses; Air popped popcorn; Peanut butter; Red wine; White wine; Water;

Herbs & Spices, Fast Foods, Prepared Foods

Cottonseed meal; Thyme (fresh); Tofu; Whole-grain cornmeal; Peppermint; Rosemary (fresh); Natto; Cheese fondue; Tempeh; Parsley; Dill weed; Spearmint (fresh); Sorghum syrup; Basil (fresh); Tarragon (dried); Succotash; French fries; Coriander/Cilantro; Fennel seeds; Oregano; Sage;

Alternative Therapies & Miscellaneous

Exposure to Sun (ten minutes per day); Follow DASH diet; Exercise; Fat-free or low fat products; Fresh (uncooked) fruits/veg's or no salt added canned; Meditation; Ornish Plan & Diet; Pray, practice your religion; Sleep 6-8 hours regularly; Tai Chi; Yoga (certain posture must be avoided); Salt-free or low-salt foods; Organically grown foods;

Key Nutrients & Herbal Medicines

Vitamin D; Hawthorn (in berries form or tea from dried leaves and flowers; do not take with other heart medications); Calcium; Celery seed; Siberian Ginseng; Magnesium; Potassium; Yucca; Boron;

Do not choose these for High Blood Pressure & Vitamin D Deficiency

Top 5 items to avoid:

Chocolate & Sweets; 2+ Alcoholic drinks/day; Cured & Luncheon Meats; Margarine & Hydrogenated vegetable oil; & Excess Body Weight

Avoid or consume much less of the following (within a food group, most harmful items are listed first):

Meat, Fish & Poultry

Frankfurters; Luncheon meats; Pepperoni; Pork liver cheese; Pork skins; Salami; Sausage; Cured meats; Pork breakfast strips; Chorizo; Cured beef; Bacon; Pastrami; Beef jerky sticks; Bologna; Chicken skin; Turkey skins; Meatless sausage; Corned beef; Pork headcheese; Salmon (smoked, Lox); Beef chuck/brisket; Pork cured/ham; Beef tongue; Squab (pigeon); Beef ribs; Lamb tongue; Lamb ribs; Beef shank;

Instead choose: Cuttlefish; Dungeness crab; Oysters; Blue crab; Cod; Beef liver; Chicken breast (no skin); Haddock; Beef/Lamb brain; Canned tuna; Orange roughy; Scallops; Pork leg/ham; Sablefish; Rabbit meat; Turkey breast; Venison; Veal shank; Veal liver; Turkey dark meat; Pork shldr; Chicken liver; Boar meat; Beef filet mignon; Beef round steak; Croaker; Pheasant; Veal; Duck (no skin); Quail breast; Ground beef; Guinea hen; Alaskan king crab; Lamb leg; Pork ribs; Beef rib eye; Lobster;

Eggs, Beans, Nuts and Seeds

Coconut milk;

Instead choose: Macadamia nuts; Egg; Coconut meat (dried); Coconut; Egg white;

Fruits & Juices

Sugared fruit Juice or made from concentrate

Instead choose: Rhubarb; Cranberries; Olives;

Vegetables

Canned vegetables;

Instead choose: Sweet potatoes

Breads, Grains, Cereals, Pasta

Saltines crackers; Croissant; Danish pastry; Wheat crackers; Sweet rolls; Milk crackers; Rice crisps cereal; Donuts; Kaiser dinner rolls; French rolls; Biscuits; White bread; Chinese chow Mein noodles;

Instead choose: Oat bran bread; Oat bran; Semolina; Pumpernickel bread; Spinach spaghetti; Corn flakes; White rice; Wheat; Corn muffins;

Dairy Products, Fats & Oils

Margarine (salted); Margarine-like spreads; Hydrogenated vegetable oil; Margarine (unsalted); Animal fats; Oils: Babassu, Cocoa Butter, cottonseed, Cupu Assu, palm, peanut, poppy seed, rice bran, sesame, Shea nut, tea seed, Ucuhuba Butter; Brie cheese; various seeds/nuts/vegetable oils; Vegetable shortening; Chocolate milk; Butter (salted); Roquefort cheese; Cheeses: goat, pimento, feta, camembert; Lard; various cheese; Cheese spread; Whipped cream; Butter (unsalted); Cream; Canola oil; Poultry fats;

Instead choose: Menhaden fish oil; Milk; Gruyere cheese; Skim milk; Yogurt; Cheddar cheese; Ricotta cheese; Colby cheese; Port de salut cheese;

Desserts, Snacks, Beverages

Chocolate ice cream; Sweet chocolate; Chocolate chip cookies; Pound cake; various cookies; Pie crust; Puff pastry; various cakes; Éclairs; Cheesecake; Coffee liqueur; Cream puffs; Pretzels; Dessert toppings; Coffee; Coffeecake; Chocolate mousse; Vanilla cream pie; Pecan pie; Hot chocolate; various pies; Fruit leather/rolls; After-dinner mints; Vanilla ice cream; Pudding; Potato sticks; Ice cream cones; Frostings; Soft (carbonated) drinks; Plain tea; Fruit punch; Lemonade; Pancakes;

Instead choose: Dark chocolate; Tonic water; Potato chips/fried snacks; Beer; Sports drinks; Milk shakes; Halvah; Eggnog; Malted drinks (nonalcoholic); Applesauce; Ginger ale; Herbal tea;

Herbs & Spices, Fast Foods, Prepared Foods

Salad dressings: Blue/Roquefort, French; Table salt; Oyster sauce; Foie gras or liver pate; Italian salad dressing; Sauces: Hoisin, Sofrito; Hot dog; Barbecue sauce; Capers; Mayonnaise; various sauces; Breaded shrimp; Soy sauce; Chicken Nuggets; Table sugar (white or powder); Chocolate syrup; Nachos; Pizza; Ketchup; Tabasco sauce; Onion rings; Hash brown potatoes; Syrup (table blends); Pickle relish; Mustard; Pickle (cucumber); Cheeseburger; Gravies (canned);

Instead choose: Tomato paste; Chervil; Poppy seed; Cayenne (red) pepper; Cinnamon; Pepper (black or white); Turmeric; Mustard seed; Falafel; Miso; Cocoa; Corn salad; Mints; Saffron; Maple sugar; Fish stock; Cardamom; Mace; Cloves; Chives; Ginger; Marjoram; Brown sugar; Vinegar; Clam chowder; Nutmeg; Minestrone soup; Beef stock; Chicken stock; Sweet pickle;

Alternative Therapies & Miscellaneous

Excess body weight; 2+ alcoholic drinks/day; Hyperthermia (avoid if extremely high blood pressure); Smoking, tobacco; Stress; Salted foods, nuts, etc.; Corn sweetener;

Key Nutrients & Herbal Medicines

Caffeine; Licorice; Sodium/salt (limit to 1,500 mg per day); Guarana; Kola (cola); Mate;

DASH Diet

DASH stands for Dietary Approaches to Stop Hypertension, and was developed by the US Department of Health and Human Services.

Based on research by the National Heart, Lung, and Blood Institute (NHLBI) the DASH eating plan lowers blood pressure.

DASH is a diet rich in fruits, vegetables and low-fat dairy foods, and low in sodium, saturated fat, cholesterol and total fat. It favors foods rich in nutrients that are expected to lower blood pressure, such as potassium, calcium, magnesium, protein, and fiber. It contains fewer sweets, added sugars, and red meats than typical American diet.

The DASH eating plan promotes foods rich in potassium, but does not recommend potassium supplements.

Reduced-sodium products and salt substitutes are not recommended either due to potential harmful effect of potassium chloride as a main ingredient.

In addition to lowering blood pressure, the DASH diet may help against other conditions including obesity, osteoporosis, cancer, heart disease, stroke and diabetes.

Choose these for DASH Diet

Top 5 items to consume:

Fish; Whole Grains/Whole-wheat; Soybeans/Soymilk; Beans/Legumes; Seeds & Nuts;

Food items and actions that could improve your health (within a food group, most helpful items are listed first):

Meat, Fish & Poultry **up to 6 oz. fish, poultry or lean meat per day**

Monkfish; Freshwater bass; Seabass; Bluefish; Burbot; Carp; Catfish; Chicken breast (no skin); Cusk; Grouper; Halibut; Ling; Lingcod; King mackerel; Marlin; Mullet; Perch; Northern pike; Pumpkinseed sunfish; Pink salmon; Sheepshead; Snapper; Spot; Sturgeon; Sucker; Swordfish; Tilapia; Tilefish; Trout; various types of tuna; White fish; Wolffish; Pout; Whiting; Walleye; Turkey breast; Pollock; Yellowtail; Mackerel; Dolphinfish (Mahi-Mahi); Shark; Drum; Scup; Milkfish; Rockfish; Cisco; Turbot; Cod; Herring; Striped bass; Pheasant; Surimi; Smelt; Butterfish; Pompano fish; Shad; Quail breast; Turkey; Orange roughy; Seatrout; Turkey dark meat; Flatfish (flounder & sole); Cisco (smoked); Guinea hen; Sardines; Haddock; Quail; Duck (no skin); White fish (smoked); Chicken wings; Chicken giblets; Chicken liver; Croaker; Cuttlefish; Turkey liver; Chicken dark meat; Turkey giblets; Sablefish; Goose; Turkey heart; Chicken heart; Snail; Whelk; Anchovy; Squab (pigeon);

Eggs, Beans, Nuts and Seeds **4-5 servings of nuts/seeds/beans per week; 1 serving = 1.5 oz. nuts; .5 oz. seeds; 1/2 cup cooked beans**

Soybean seeds; Alfalfa sprouts; Almonds; various beans; Brazil nuts; Breadfruit seeds; Butternuts; Cashew nuts; Chestnuts; Chickpeas; Ginkgo nuts; Hazelnuts or Filberts; Lentils; Lupin; Peanuts; various types of peas; Pine nuts; Pistachio nuts; various types of seeds; Soy milk; Soybeans (green); Walnuts; Acorns; Lima beans; Pili nuts; Beechnuts; Hickory nuts; Pecans; Cornnuts; Macadamia nuts; Coconut;

Fruits & Juices **4-5 servings/day; 1 serving = 1/2 cup fruit or juice; 1 med size fruit; 1/4 cup dried fruit**

Dried fruits: Apricots, Banana, Currants; Dates; dried figs; Goji berry; Dried: Litchi, Peaches, Prunes; Raisins; Tamarind; dried Longans; Passion fruit; Dried: Pears, Apples; Elderberries; Abiyuch; Banana; Guava; Prune juice; Durian; Plantains; Pineapple juice; Blackberries; Boysenberries; Breadfruit; Currants (raw); Grape juice; Kiwi fruit; Kumquats; various berries; Rowal; Cranberry juice; Pears; Apricots; Cantaloupe; Figs; Jujube (fruit); Lemon; Lime; Longans; Natal Plum (Carissa); Persimmons; Pomegranate; Apple juice; Grapefruit juice; Orange juice; Avocado; Apples; Grapes; Peaches; Acerola; Cherries; Grapefruit; Honeydew melon; Litchi; Mango; Nectarine; Oranges; Papaya; Pineapple; Pitanga; Plum; Pomegranate juice; Pumelo (Shaddock); Quince; Strawberries; Tangerines; Watermelon; Cranberries; Rhubarb; Olives;

Vegetables **4-5 servings/day; 1 serving = 1/2 cup cut-up or juice; 1 cup leafy raw vegetables**

Balsam pear leafy tips; Epazote; Fungi cloud ears; Grape leaves; Shitake mushrooms; Ancho & pasilla peppers; Pigeon peas; Sweet potatoes leaves; Sun-dried tomatoes; Wasabi root; Amaranth leaves; Taro leaves; Artichoke; Garlic; Arrowhead; Chrysanthemum (Garland); Chrysanthemum Leaves; Dandelion Greens; Mustard spinach; Vine spinach (Basella); Tahitian taro; Potatoes w/skin; Garden cress; Kale; Taro; Collards; Mustard greens; Okra; Turnip greens; Winged beans leaves; Yam; Arugula; Chinese broccoli; Chicory greens; Kelp; Nopal; Shallots; Lotus root; Quinoa seed; Bok choy; Broccoli; Brussels sprouts; Cowpeas leafy tips; Kohlrabi; Parsnips; Balsam pear; Borage; Carrots; Endive; Fennel; Green onions (scallions); Purslane; Watercress; Hot chili peppers; Cauliflower; various peppers; Arrowroot; Portabella mushrooms; Savoy cabbage; Squash; Zucchini; Jerusalem artichoke; Beets; Green cabbage; Celery; Celtuce; Eggplant; Fiddlehead ferns; Green beans; Rutabaga; Potato; Bell peppers; Red cabbage; Leeks; Jew's ear mushrooms; other vegetables;

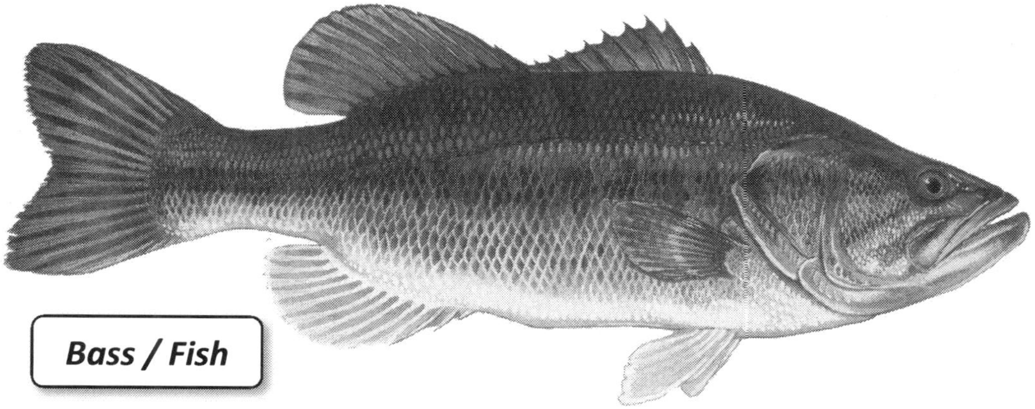

Bass / Fish

Breads, Grains, Cereals, Pasta **6-8 servings of whole-grains per day. 1 serving = 1 slice of bread; 1/2 cup cooked rice/pasta**

Wheat bran; Wheat germ; Whole-wheat; Amaranth; Whole-wheat bread; Buckwheat; Whole-wheat cereal; Corn bran; Durum wheat; Oats; Rye; Sorghum; Whole-wheat spaghetti; Triticale; Whole-wheat English muffins; Wheat germ cereal; Spelt (cooked); Oatmeal (cereal); Brown rice; Millet; Barley; Bulgur; Corn; Wild rice; Rice bran; Whole-wheat dinner rolls; Wheat germ bread; Shredded wheat cereal; Wheat bran muffins; Bran flakes cereal; Whole-wheat crackers; Oat bran muffins; Tortillas (corn);

Dairy Products, Fats & Oils **Low fat dairy: 2-3 servings/day; 1 serving= 1 cup milk or yogurt; 1.5 Oz. cheese**

Skim milk; Whey (dried); Cottage cheese; other milk; Yogurt; Chocolate milk; Swiss cheese; Ricotta cheese; Fat-free or Low Fat products

Desserts, Snacks, Beverages

Air-popped Popcorn; Milk shakes; Water;

Herbs & Spices, Fast Foods, Prepared Foods

Whole-grain Cornmeal; Cottonseed meal; Thyme (fresh); Tofu; Cocoa; Chicken stock; Natto; Rosemary (fresh); Peppermint; Chicken broth; Chicken noodle soup; Fried tofu; Tempeh; Spearmint (fresh); Parsley;

Alternative Therapies & Miscellaneous

Fat-free or low fat products; Fresh (uncooked) fruits/veg's or no salt added canned;

Key Nutrients & Herbal Medicines

Calcium; Fiber; Magnesium; Potassium; Protein;

<u>Do not</u> choose these for DASH Diet

Top 5 items to avoid:

Sweets & Sugar; Cured & Luncheon Meats; Margarine; Salad dressings & Sauces; Animal fats;

Avoid or consume much less of the following (within a food group, most harmful items are listed first):

Meat, Fish & Poultry

Cured meats; Bacon; Cured beef; Beerwurst beer salami; Chorizo; Frankfurters; Luncheon meats; Pepperoni; Pork liver cheese; Pork skins; Salamis; Sausages; Pastrami; Bologna; Beef jerky sticks; Caviar; Pork cured/ham; Pork headcheese; Lamb/Beef tongue; Meatless sausage; Shrimp; Corned beef; Lamb/Pork/Beef ribs; Beef chuck/brisket; Beef/Lamb brain; Calamari; Ground lamb; Clams; Lobster; Pancreas (lamb, beef, veal); Pork spare ribs; Veal tongue; Alaskan king crab; Beef shank; Lamb heart; Pork/Veal lungs; Lamb loin; Lamb shoulder; Abalone; Pork shldr;

Instead <u>choose</u>: Octopus; Salmon (smoked, Lox); Spiny lobster; Boar meat; Venison; Fish roe; Beef filet mignon; Pork loin/sirloin; Mussels; Rabbit meat; Beef round steak; Veal shank; Dungeness crab; Beef liver; Ground beef; Scallops; Veal loin; Crayfish; Eel; Beef rib eye; Oysters; Blue crab; Veal liver; Lamb leg; Pork leg/ham;

Eggs, Beans, Nuts and Seeds **Limit to 4 egg yolks per week**

Egg yolk; Coconut milk; Egg substitute; Egg;

Fruits & Juices

Sugared fruit Juice or made from concentrate;

Breads, Grains, Cereals, Pasta

Croissant; Saltines crackers; Sweet rolls; Wheat crackers; Danish pastry; Milk crackers; Donuts; Biscuits; Rice crisps cereal; Waffles; Kaiser dinner rolls; French rolls; Blueberry muffins; Hamburger & hot dog rolls; Chinese chow Mein noodles; Granola bars; Melba toasts crackers; White bread; Corn flakes;

Instead <u>choose</u>: Semolina; Rice cakes (Brown rice based); Wheat; Oat bran bread; Oat bran; Granola cereal; Spinach spaghetti; Pumpernickel bread; Japanese noodles; Spaghetti; White rice; Egg noodles; Couscous; Rice noodles; Pasta; English muffins; Cream of wheat; Italian bread;

Dairy Products, Fats & Oils

limit to 2-3 servings of fats & oils/day; 1 serving = 1 tsp. margarine or veg oil; 1 Tbsp. mayo or salad dressing

Margarine (salted); Margarine-like spreads; Animal fat; Lard; Butter (salted); Margarine (unsalted); Oils: Babassu, Cocoa Butter, coconut, corn, cottonseed, Cupu Assu; Hydrogenated vegetable oil; various seeds/nuts/vegetable oils; Vegetable shortening; various fish oils; Butter (unsalted); Cheeses: American, Roquefort, pimento; Cod liver fish oil; Cheeses: feta, Brie, cream, blue, camembert; Cheese spread; Cheeses: parmesan, limburger; Non-dairy creamers;

Instead choose: Gruyere cheese; Sour cream; Wheat germ oil; Cheeses: Gjetost, Mozzarella, Colby, Cheddar, Port de salut;

Desserts, Snacks, Beverages

limit to 5 or less servings of sweets per week; 1 serving=1 Tbsp. sugar/jelly/jam; 1/2 cup sorbet or gelatin; 1 cup lemonade

After-dinner mints; Cakes; Candies; Sweet chocolate; Cheesecake; Chocolate mousse; Dark chocolate; Coffeecake; Cookies; Cream puffs; Dessert toppings; Éclairs; Frostings; Ice cream cones; Ice creams; Pancakes; various pies; Puff pastry; Chewing gum; Jams & Preserves; Sherbet; Fruit leather/rolls; Jellies; Pudding; Fruit punch; Lemonade; Honey; Pretzels; Soft (carbonated) drinks; Potato sticks; Frozen yogurt; Coffee liqueur; 80+ proof distilled alc. bev.; Whiskey; Taro chips; Crème de menthe; Potato chips/fried snacks; Piña colada; Tortilla chips;

Instead choose: Tonic water; Plain tea; Hot chocolate; Peanut butter; sports drinks; Coffee; Applesauce; Ginger ale; Herbal tea; Oil popped popcorn; Malted drinks (nonalcoholic); Green tea;

Herbs & Spices, Fast Foods, Prepared Foods

Various salad dressings; Oyster sauce; Table sugar (white or powder); Hoisin sauce; Table salt; Chocolate syrup; Soy sauce; various sauces; Barbecue sauce; Capers; Syrup (table blends); Hot dog; Mayonnaise; Breaded shrimp; Nachos; Maple syrup; Onion rings; Ketchup; Pizza; Tabasco sauce; Malt syrup; Teriyaki sauce; Foie gras or liver pate; Hash brown potatoes; Potato pancakes; Potato salad; Pickle relish; Mustard; Hush puppies; French toast; Pickle (cucumber); Cheeseburger; Sorghum syrup; Gravies (canned); Tapioca; Sauerkraut; Taco shells; Macaroni; Miso;

Instead choose: Dill weed; Succotash; Cheese fondue; Basil (fresh); Coriander/Cilantro; Oregano; Sage; Tarragon (dried); Fennel seeds; Chervil; Beef stock; Cayenne (red) pepper; Pepper (black or white); Turmeric; Mustard seed; Cinnamon; French fries; Poppy seed; Corn salad; Saffron; Molasses; Cardamom; Mace; Mints; Maple sugar; Fish stock; Chives; Ginger; Marjoram; Brown sugar; Vinegar; Falafel; Beef broth; Veg/beef soup; Nutmeg; Tomato paste; Cloves;

Alternative Therapies & Miscellaneous

Corn sweetener; Salted foods, nuts, etc.; 2+ alcoholic drinks/day; Processed or Refined foods; Baking using butter; Fried or battered foods; Smoking, tobacco; Salt-free or low-salt foods (due to harmful effects of potassium chloride ingredient);

Key Nutrients & Herbal Medicines

Sodium/salt (up to 2,300 mg/day; preferably less than 1,500 mg/day); Refined Sugar; Alcohol; Cholesterol; Saturated fat; Total fat;

References

All the material and suggestions presented in this book are based on the content available at PersonalRemedies.com. The primary sources used by that web site and therefore this book are US government sources such as:

- USDA (US Department of Agriculture) including USDA Dietary Guidelines for Americans, nutrition.gov and mypyramid.gov.
- NIH (National Institute of Health) including Office of Dietary Supplements (ods.od.nih.gov), and MedlinePlus Health Information – a service of National Library of Medicine and NIH, National Diabetes Information Clearinghouse (NDIC), National Heart, Lung and Blood Institute ...
- Other organizations such as: Centers for Disease Control and Prevention (cdc.gov), National Cancer Institute (cancer.gov), US Environmental Protection Agency ...

For complete and detailed information about all the references please visit PersonalRemedies.com.

For Additional Information

For personal food list suggestions for

- other health conditions,
- other combinations of health conditions,
- a greater list of food choices, and
- for more detailed nutritional information,

you may wish to look at other books in our *Choose this not that* series listed on the last page or visit PersonalRemedies.com.

Acknowledgements

We would like to thank the following individuals for their support, encouragement, advice and contributions to the production of this book and contents of the Personal Remedies knowledgebase which is presented in this book: Ester Awnetwant-Esperon, MS, RD, LD; Karen Chiacu-Recco; Kate Fletcher-King; Amanda King; Avirat Kulkarni; Barbara Langathianos; Andrew Lenhardt, MD; Sih Han Lim; Mark Lu, MD; Steve Manson; Art McCray; Dick Neville; Christian Seeber; Nancy Elizabeth Shaw; Diana Silk; Scott Silk; George Sprenkle; Shahin Tabatabaei, MD; Foad Vafaei; Rolie Zagnoli; Mory Bahar.

Personal Remedies, LLC

and

Simple Software Publishing

Who is Personal Remedies?

Personal Remedies is a leading provider of knowledgebase & software for nutrition and health. The company can enable organizations such as hospitals, clinics, physician groups, food retailers, weight loss companies, leading fitness organizations, mobile phone operators and progressive corporations to provide consumer-centric nutrition, diet and health information tailored to the unique profile and goals of an individual.

Who is Simple Software Publishing?

Simple Software Publishing is a small publisher established in 1996. Our passion is to explain complex matters in an easy to understand form. We also strive to minimize the use of paper for production and distribution of books.

Choose this not that Series of Books, eBooks and Apps

- *Choose this not that* for **Breast Cancer**
- *Choose this not that* for **Cancer Prevention**
- *Choose this not that* for **Cervical Cancer**
- *Choose this not that* for **Colon Cancer**
- *Choose this not that* for **Esophageal Cancer**
- *Choose this not that* for **Gout**
- *Choose this not that* for **High Blood Pressure**
- *Choose this not that* for **High Cholesterol**
- *Choose this not that* for **High Triglycerides**
- *Choose this not that* for **Lung Cancer**
- *Choose this not that* for **Ovarian Cancer**
- *Choose this not that* for **Pancreatic Cancer**
- *Choose this not that* for **Prostate Cancer**
- *Choose this not that* for **Rheumatoid Arthritis**
- *Choose this not that* for **Stomach Cancer**
- *Choose this not that* for **Ulcers**
- *Choose this not that* for **Vitamin D Deficiency**
- *Choose this not that* for … **please send us your suggestion!**

How to Order

To order eBooks (on Kindle or Nook) or printed copies of this book, or to order any of our other books please visit Amazon.com, Barnes & Noble, or contact us by email at Publisher@PersonalRemedies.com or send your purchase order or payments to:

Simple Software Publishing
5 Oregon Street
Georgetown, MA 01833

To order a colorful Mobile App version of this book, please visit Google Play Store (Android), or visit Amazon App Store.

For suggestions for new books and comments please email us at Books@PersonalRemedies.com.

Progress Tracker

To monitor your progress, date and note your symptoms and relevant data such as blood pressure, weight, cholesterol level ... below. We love to hear about your feedback and progress. Email us at Books@PersonalRemedies.com.

Notes

Made in the USA
Middletown, DE
29 November 2025

23514904R00062